Praise for Paint Your Hair Blue

"A heartbreaking yet heartwarming story of how Taylor and her family navigated pediatric cancer with love, laughter, and tears. Beautifully written, it feels as if you're going through the journey with Taylor and her family. *Paint Your Hair Blue* will make you hug your children tighter and fight harder to find a cure for pediatric cancer."

–Angie Harmon, mother, actress, director, UNICEF Ambassador

"*Paint Your Hair Blue* is a heartwarming memoir that uncovers the battles a strong and beautiful young girl fought through as a pediatric cancer patient. As a parent, I cannot imagine the pain that Taylor's parents endured and greatly admire their courage to share this incredible story of love and perseverance-a poignant reminder to both live life and love others to our greatest capacity."

–Hannah Storm ESPN award-winning journalist

"If you've ever loved someone with all your strength, mind, heart, and soul, this book–this love story–will appeal to you. The author tells a deeply personal story about her young daughter's determination to stay alive despite the onslaught of pediatric cancer. Your heart will break and soar, sometimes simultaneously, as you learn about Taylor's fierce courage and unremitting resolve to not permit cancer to scar her spirit along with her body. As much as any drug or medical protocol, readers quickly realize that Taylor's best medicine, and the one that worked better than any other, was the lavish and unconditional love of her father, mother, and sisters.

"*Paint Your Hair Blue* is a mother's longing to give enduring eloquence to a daughter's voice, to not let it go silent. Readers will come away from the book with a vivid understanding of how truly short and precious life is and a greater willingness to add more color as we go along."

–Reverend Anthony Penna, B

"Taylor's was a life worth living, and this is a book well worth reading. *Paint Your Hair Blue* is an inspiring memoir about a laughing, fun-loving teen who lived life on her own terms despite having cancer. This book will resonate with anyone going through a difficult diagnosis. Filled with anecdotes that will help you survive the medical world, it is a love story that will have you shaking your head about the state of pediatric oncology as well as the grace and determination of one little warrior."

–Nancy Taddiken, retired superintendent for Edgemont Schools,
Taylor's friend and hero

Paint Your Hair Blue

Paint Your Hair Blue

A Celebration of Life with Hope for Tomorrow in the Face of PEDIATRIC CANCER

A MEMOIR

Sue Matthews

with her sister Andrea Cohane

NEW YORK

LONDON • NASHVILLE • MELBOURNE • VANCOUVER

Paint Your Hair *Blue*

*A Celebration of Life with Hope for Tomorrow
in the Face of Pediatric Cancer*

Published in New York, New York, by Morgan James Publishing. Morgan James is a trademark of Morgan James, LLC. www.MorganJamesPublishing.com

The Morgan James Speakers Group can bring authors to your live event. For more information or to book an event visit The Morgan James Speakers Group at www.TheMorganJamesSpeakersGroup.com.

Authors have received permission to use any real names that appear in this book. All others are pseudonyms to protect privacy.

ISBN 9781683507277 paperback
ISBN 9781683507284 eBook
Library of Congress Control Number: 2017912849

Cover Design by:
Rachel Lopez
www.r2cdesign.com

Interior Design by:
Chris Treccani
www.3dogcreative.net

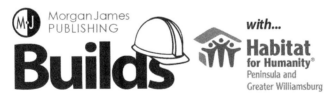

In an effort to support local communities, raise awareness and funds, Morgan James Publishing donates a percentage of all book sales for the life of each book to Habitat for Humanity Peninsula and Greater Williamsburg.

Get involved today! Visit
www.MorganJamesBuilds.com

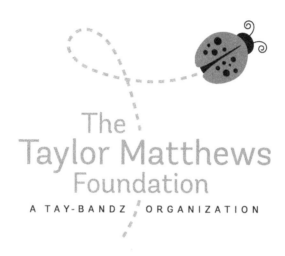

The
Taylor Matthews
Foundation

A TAY-BANDZ ORGANIZATION

A portion of the authors' proceeds from the sale of this book
will be donated to the Taylor Matthews Foundation

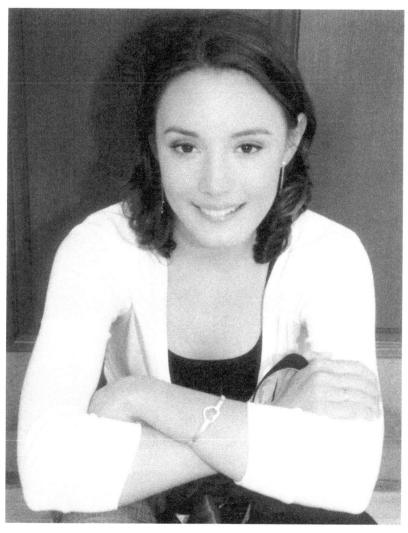

In Loving Memory of Taylor

Table of Contents

To my family, with all my love

Taylor
Thank you for showing me the true meaning of love and life
Our eternal love has no boundaries

Bob
Thank you for unconditionally loving me and breathing life into me
You are my everything

Ryan and Corey
Your love fills my heart with joy and my days with sunshine
I love you forever and always

Andrea
You encouraged me, guided me, and wrote from your heart
Your love for Taylor and us is reflected in your words

Introduction

You will find as you look back on your life, that the moments you really lived are the moments after you have done things in the spirit of love.

–Henry Drummond

Our daughter, Taylor, lost her battle with cancer when she was sixteen years old. Was Taylor's cancer journey successful? I dare say YES! How could I, as a mother, possibly say this when she ultimately lost her battle? It's not just because she beat tremendous odds and lived almost five years after her initial diagnosis. And it's not just because she made even the most jaded oncologists believe she would make it.

Taylor's cancer journey was successful because she lived every single day she had on this earth to the fullest. She lived in the moment. When she was feeling well, she was living well: laughing, playing, *and experiencing life*. I didn't teach her to do this; she taught me. What she imparted to me can apply to everyone, no matter what the prognosis or situation. Once we discovered that the most important part of Taylor's cancer journey, the day-to-day experience of it, was *in our control*, it empowered us in a way that made all the difference.

There's no way for anyone to completely avoid the fear and concomitant pain that comes along with a cancer diagnosis, but Taylor's fearless approach and insistence on living life on her own terms allowed her to live with meaning and purpose. Had Taylor abandoned her zest for life and allowed herself to become a victim, she would have cheated herself from some of her life's greatest moments and adventures, including traveling, falling in love, and just being a kid. She always found a reason to be happy, a reason to laugh, a reason to love, and a reason to live. She truly believed that all you need in life is love. Whenever I face even the slightest hardship today, I can hear her saying, "Come on; get with the program. Life sucks; wear a helmet!" And I can't help but smile.

Whether you are facing a life-threatening disease, have a loved one who is, or are just going through the normal ups and downs of life, I hope Taylor's story will give you hope, inspiration, and courage.

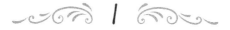

Cancer?

*You never know how strong you are until being strong
is the only choice you have.*

–Cayla Mills

Flowers Because It's Tuesday

On a bright, beautiful, atypically warm May weekend in 2003, my husband Bob and I, along with our daughters, were excited about our vacation in London, celebrating our eighteenth wedding anniversary. I have always loved to travel and see life through others' eyes, especially my children's. After three daughters, our wedding anniversary had become a family affair, as had Valentine's Day and every other holiday symbolizing love.

Bob and I met early in our college careers at Franklin & Marshall, and I was smitten from the start. His good looks, thick ink-black hair with eyes to match, Cupid's bow lips, and chiseled body had me the first time our eyes met, even if I didn't let on. There was plenty of flirting and sophomoric wooing. He constantly invited me to fraternity parties, which I ignored because he had a long-term high school romance that lingered in an "on-again, off-again" cycle, and he was firmly loyal during their "on" cycles. Sarcastically, I would laugh and engage but also send the message that I wasn't falling for any slick or sassy approaches.

Bob was undaunted. Whenever he was "single" or just a little drunk, he was pretty creative about keeping my attention. In one now-infamous story, while his fraternity hosted a Polynesian-themed party on a cold, autumn night, he walked several blocks to my apartment with one rum drink in each hand, wearing only a grass skirt and lei. After sneaking down the alley, he crouched below the windows of my first-floor apartment and positioned himself directly under my kitchen window, where he could hear that I was talking with someone. At the first lull in conversation, he sprang up into my view, bare chested and amused at my initially horrified look. I rolled my eyes, waved my hand, and casually remarked, "Oh, that's just Bob." I let him in, we shared the drinks, and then I sent him packing. I said afterwards he was definitely cute, but "immature and irresponsible."

Eventually Bob won my heart, and soon we became inseparable. By the mid-1980s, we were newlyweds, just out of college, pursuing the yuppie dream in an Upper-East-Side Manhattan apartment with a plush white rug, a balcony just large enough for two people to share a glass of wine, and a refrigerator containing little more than a jar of mustard and some instant coffee. We were both working long hours, Bob at a brokerage house and myself at a Big Four accounting firm. We were enjoying life as only twenty-somethings can, naïve and innocent, our stories yet untold but holding all the potential in the world.

When our first daughter, Ryan, was born in 1989, playgroups, arts and crafts, baking cookies, and *Sesame Street* soon consumed my days. Two years later, our second daughter, Taylor, was born. After our third daughter, Corey, was born in 1994, we settled into our dream suburban home with a white picket fence—literally. The iconic American symbolism was not lost on me. Three beautiful little girls and my Prince Charming, who, being a true romantic, would often send me roses just because it was a Tuesday.

The rest of that decade was defined, for me, by being a mother: bear hugs, Barbie dolls, kissing "boo-boos," and mending little broken hearts. Back then, my worst problem was negotiating whose turn it was to sit on Mommy's lap. Although those days were tiring, I cherished them. I loved listening to my girls' giggles or seeing the wonder in their eyes as they discovered a new toy or a frosted pink cupcake. My days were filled with peanut-butter kisses, finger paint, and tender moments of pure, unconditional love. I couldn't have asked for more.

However—and this is the strange part—I couldn't totally embrace my life. I felt *too* blessed. I had a sense of foreboding, waiting for the proverbial other shoe to drop. I just never thought it would be one of my kids.

I certainly had no real worries in May 2003 during our eighteenth wedding anniversary celebration: Ryan, Taylor, and Corey were ages thirteen, eleven, and eight. When we arrived in London, everyone was ready for a fun-filled weekend.

That first evening, we donned fancy dresses and headed out to see *Mamma Mia!* I remember sitting in the theater, looking at Bob with a big smile on my face, my eyes glowing from within, telling him with an affectionate glance how proud I was at all we had accomplished in our eighteen years together. The curtain rose. After reading so many wonderful reviews, I wasn't surprised at how much the girls were enjoying *Mamma Mia!* ABBA's bubbly and boisterous music sets in motion a love story involving a mother and her many suitors from years past. Her daughter, Mia, on the eve of her own wedding, longs to learn the identity of her real father. Her mother won't reveal his name, or maybe she doesn't know, so she narrows it down to three suitors from her past and invites them all to the wedding.

At the end of the first act, my little one, Corey turned to me with a furrowed brow. "Mommy, how could she not know who her father is? I don't understand." Ryan and Taylor burst into laughter, as any adolescents might. Adamantly, and with a bright-red face, all I could muster was, "Okay, everyone, go get a drink and leave Corey and me alone!"

When each of the girls had asked how a baby was made before they were old enough to really know, we told them, "Daddy plants a seed in Mommy," which they literally thought meant a seed in our vegetable garden. Now, Corey was about to find out the truth in the middle of intermission in a crowded London theater. In a monotone voice, I explained it to her, as scientifically as I could. Her response was, "That's just gross!" When the rest of them returned, with a stern glance I sent a silent message to Ryan and Taylor to stop whispering, snickering, and staring at Corey, but it was hard for them to resist. I admit I thought it was funny, too.

The next day, we enjoyed an afternoon shopping at our favorite store, Harrods, known for the latest fashion trends. While waiting in the shoe department, out of the blue, Taylor asked urgently, "Can I get highlights in my hair?"

"Absolutely not," I snapped, rolling my eyes. "You're eleven years old! Your hair is pristine and beautiful; you don't need to put dye in it. There's plenty of time when you're older."

None of us could have known what was lurking just around the bend, waiting to strike our family like a cyclone and wreak havoc on our world. How was I ever to know what that question and my answer would end up meaning?

Never a Dull Moment

From the day Taylor was born, she was full of spirit and sass. When the nurses handed her to Bob and me for the first time, I expected to see a beautiful baby with supple skin, sweet and soft. Instead, her face was covered with red, raw, deep scratches. Amused, the doctor explained, "Taylor probably scratched her face in the womb, willing herself to come into the world of the living!" We laughed along with him, but we had no idea how typical this type of feisty behavior would prove to be. With Taylor, there was never a dull moment.

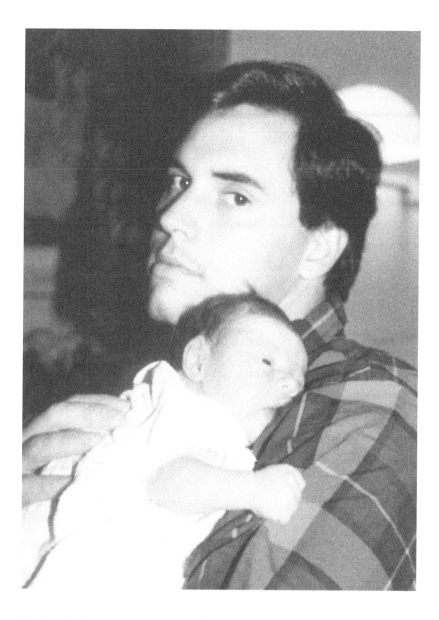

Taylor didn't experience the terrible twos, but the terrible twos, threes, and fours. Whenever she misbehaved, which was quite often and typically included taunting her older sister Ryan, she was given a "time out" and told to go to her room. Taylor was never going to do things anyone else's way. Telling her she had to do something was a sure way to make sure she didn't.

During time out, she refused to stay in her room, slowly inching out to the hallway until she stood right in front of me. I couldn't control her. She would smile and say, "Mammie, I a good girrrl now." The only punishment that ever worked was my refusal to speak to her. She would cry, "I lovvve you, Mammie. I am sawry."

Although Taylor could be a smart-alecky little pest, she was so lovable it was hard to stay angry. Her passion for life was contagious. Little things excited her, and she could make even the dullest cloudy day appear exquisite, if you just looked at it through her eyes. She was irresistible even on her worst day, and she knew it, sometimes taking full advantage of us. When she bestowed her love upon you, you felt like the most important person in the world.

We all thought she looked like a younger version of the actress Natalie Portman, but she was much happier to say that she resembled me. She was small boned, with light olive skin; a straight nose; long, pin-straight, shiny brown hair; and, most beguiling, a mischievous smile that accentuated her full red lips.

Taylor's due date was November 4, too close for comfort to my older sister Lynn's birthday, November 8. I hadn't wanted Taylor to share her birthday with Lynn. Although Lynn is a brunette like me and strangers sometimes can't tell us apart, on the inside we couldn't be more different. She is extremely volatile and self-absorbed. It could take an entire book to tell Lynn's story; quite frankly, it's not worth the ink. Suffice it to say, Lynn wasn't speaking to me on either the day Taylor was born or on the day she died. Since Taylor's funeral, neither she nor her daughters have spoken to me or my other sister, Andrea. She cut us both off and has flat-out refused to give an explanation.

Despite the bad blood, Taylor shared one characteristic with her aunt. Like Lynn, Taylor was known for what we called her "otherworldliness" and could relay countless stories about her premonitions. My dearest friend Janet, whom I can confide in about anything, has always agreed that Taylor had a mystical way about her, a sixth sense, a knowing beyond the rest of us. She had an aura that transcended her physical presence and an understanding of life beyond her years.

Taylor's most shocking premonition came on September 10, 2001, the night before 9/11, when she kept me up the entire night insisting, "Mommy, something horrible is going to happen tomorrow." Disbelieving, I replied to my nine-year-old, "You're crazy. Go to sleep!" I figured it was one more of Taylor's notorious nighttime woes.

No matter what I said, nothing calmed her down. She simply wouldn't let up. We cuddled all night as I tried to assuage her fears. The following day, one that no American will ever forget, Taylor came home from school with anger in her eyes. She folded her arms and said, "See! I told you so." I was stunned.

Even when Taylor wasn't predicting the future, her imagination ran wild. She dreamed about alien abductions and was often concocting a mischievous scheme, whether it was climbing a tree or pulling a prank. She especially reveled in teasing her little sister, Corey. One time she neatly pasted decorative, blue glue dots across a page of paper. She then enthusiastically told Corey to "hurry up and eat them; they're the old-fashioned candy dots on paper that Mommy never lets us have." Corey fell for it, just as she did when Taylor pulled a similar prank with a "sweet" jalapeno pepper. Needless to say, all of her antics ended with Corey in tears and Taylor in hysterics. A dear friend of Taylor's, Becca, put it perfectly years later: "Taylor has the maturity level of an eight-year-old boy!"

At eleven, Taylor was extremely energetic, with chubby cheeks often rosy from exertion on the playground. She never sat still; her mind and body were always galloping. The word "rest" simply did not exist in Taylor's vocabulary. As far as I was concerned, she was the picture of health; she had never even been on an antibiotic in her life.

Soccer was one of Taylor's passions, although more for the camaraderie between her and her teammates than for the sport itself. She wasn't the best athlete on the team, but she put in 150 percent every time. It was all for fun, for helping the team, win or lose.

That spring, she began experiencing some shortness of breath during soccer practice, so just to be safe, I scheduled an appointment with her pediatrician shortly before we set off for the anniversary trip to London. After examining her, our pediatrician diagnosed Taylor with exercise-induced asthma and gave me a handful of prescriptions, so many they filled a large Ziploc bag. I thought to myself, *Why would I give Taylor all this medicine before consulting a specialist?* I certainly wasn't worried about anything serious; I was being cautious, as is my nature. When I spoke to my pediatrician about seeing a pulmonologist, she insisted, "You're totally overreacting. Her lungs are clear." I responded harshly, "I want expert advice on her medication doses, and I want her to blow in the box. Period." I walked out as the doctor rolled her eyes at my "overreaction."

Upon our return from London, Taylor was scheduled to see a pulmonologist so we could get her asthma medicine sorted. She was especially excited on the day of her appointment because at school they were receiving bunk assignments for sixth grade camp, a five-day overnight school trip that most kids look forward to from kindergarten. I picked her up midday from school, intending to bring her back after our appointment.

"Leave your backpack in your cubby, sweetheart. You'll be back in less than two hours."

"Mommy, my teacher is mad that I left during orientation to sixth grade camp."

"It's fine," I reminded her. "You have a doctor's appointment, and I signed you out."

"But Mommy, she is *pissed*."

"Tales, do we really care if she's pissed at you?" I chortled as we exchanged broad, knowing grins. Even then I knew better than to worry about nonsense.

While driving to the pulmonologist, Taylor was like a little kid on a long road trip, asking over and over, "How long will it take?"

I finally asked, "What's up, Tales?"

"I need to be back for recess because I have a lot to plan for sixth grade camp with Jenny."

Jenny, a cutie pie with golden blonde hair and a hop in her step, was Taylor's best friend, and they were a perfect match, mischievous, fun loving, and full of *chutzpah*. "I have to get back!" she insisted. I couldn't help smiling to myself. She then added with pure excitement, "And, plus Mommy, it's Thursday!" Soccer practice day.

Shortly after our arrival at the doctor's office, the pulmonologist ordered a routine chest x-ray and then had Taylor breathe into tubes to measure her oxygen output. I could see Taylor's devilish grin; she knew she was doing well. She announced, "I like this doctor, Mommy. I know he's going to make me better."

As the pulmonologist examined her, I began making a list of what I needed to pack for sixth grade camp. Just that morning I had bought bells to hang on Taylor's bed to alert the teachers in case Taylor awoke in the middle of the night. Even at night, Taylor didn't stay still. She was a boisterous sleepwalker. I grimaced, remembering the night she came into our room and woke us up chanting, "Where is my guitar; where is it?" Bob and I knew we had to play along with her story, or else she would become very confrontational. Taylor never had a guitar or any interest in playing one, but she always had an interesting tale to tell while she was sleepwalking.

Suddenly, the doctor interrupted my reverie and in a flat voice asked, "Mrs. Matthews, can you come upstairs to my office?" I asked Taylor, "Are you comfortable with that?" She frowned but said, "Fine," rolling her eyes and not hiding her disapproval. Gathering my belongings, I casually got up from my chair and made my way to his office. In the elevator, I inquired, "Could this be serious?" After a pregnant pause, the doctor shocked me by responding, "Maybe."

I walked into his office; oddly, I felt a slight shift in the air and a sense of sadness. *What could be wrong,* I wondered, with a sick feeling in the pit of my stomach. Then the doctor showed me Taylor's chest x-ray. The only x-ray I had ever seen was of Ryan's broken wrist years ago, but when I saw this, even I knew it was *bad*. Taylor's lungs were filled with little white spots, irregular in size, and near her ribs was a large, white spot about the size of a plum. I trembled. I remember looking at my watch, noting it was 12:19 p.m.

At that moment, I somehow comprehended, knowing as little as I did, that life as I knew it was over. Shaking, I murmured, "Is this cancer?" He replied hastily with many alternative explanations, but I wanted a straight answer. This would be my first of many confrontations with the medical world. In a high-pitched voice I didn't recognize as my own, I shrieked, "Do I need to call my husband?" All he could muster was, "Yes, Mrs. Matthews. You should call him right away."

Bob was with one of his newest advisors, helping him with a large opportunity that could be a game changer for him and the entire brokerage branch Bob ran. They were poised to give a presentation they had been working on for a long time, and Bob was more than a little nervous. As they were approaching security in a downtown Manhattan building, his cell phone rang.

"Bob, it's me," I managed to say, shaking, barely able to hold the telephone up to my ear. The minute he heard my voice he knew something was very wrong.

"What's going on?"

"I'm at the doctor's office. It's Taylor. The doctor says she might have cancer." As I whispered those words, my heart palpitated so quickly I thought I might faint. As I waited for his response, it felt as if my entire life was flashing before me.

Oddly, Bob remembers my words differently. He remembers hearing, "The x-ray shows a bunch of spots on her lungs. They think this is serious." He doesn't recall me ever saying the word "cancer." Most likely, neither of us will ever know the first words we exchanged, but we both know he responded with urgency, "I'm on the way."

He caught the first cab to Grand Central Terminal and the first train to Edgemont, our hometown, to get his car, and then raced to the hospital. He tried to think of explanations that would make everything okay, praying and bargaining with God. *God, if you let T be okay, I'll become a better person, dedicate myself to charity, drop all bad habits, you name it.* In time, we would both learn there is no bargaining with God.

It probably took him two hours to get to the doctor's office. I was drowning inside, but I willed myself to stay calm and not let my fear reverberate through to Taylor.

The doctor had ordered a CT scan. Apparently if you have exercise-induced asthma, you must first drink "contrast" before the scan and come back the next day, so the nurse was refusing to give Taylor the scan. I remember throwing up my arms in a fury and belting out, "Please! Just call the doctor!" I overheard the doctor tell the nurse, "Follow normal protocol; she doesn't have exercise-induced asthma." BAM! It hit me again. She probably has *cancer*, a concept I couldn't grasp.

The lights in the scan room were obnoxiously bright, almost as if they were trying to irritate me, but despite the light, my vision became dim, fuzzy, and unreliable. My limbs felt heavy, my heart was racing, and I wanted to scream out in horror. Instead, I simply looked at Taylor and smiled. Taylor leaned her head on my shoulder and, with a deep sigh and fire in her eyes, said as loudly as she could, "Mommy, I'm *starving*! Do I really have to take this stupid test? Can't we just get lunch now?"

Food was always of the utmost importance to Taylor, and she hated my cooking, many times throwing a fit and refusing to eat it. She was often in trouble as a tyke as a result, and she was known for her letters of apology afterwards. One of her funnier apology letters reads, "Mommy, I'm sorry I wouldn't eat dinner tonight. But, next time could you maybe try some barbeque sauce? And by the way, while I was writing this note, you came in and yelled at me again."

When Taylor was placed in the scanner, I was finally alone and able to make a call without her hearing. Bob had not yet arrived. I called my soul mate, my sister Andrea, who affectionately lets us—and I mean only us—call her Annie. She is the youngest of my three siblings, ten years my junior. Andrea is a petite, smart, and a feisty blonde who claims she is 5 feet 1 and 1/4 inches tall and whose exuberance could brighten anyone's day. She looks nothing like me, her dark-haired, dark-eyed sister, but our hearts were one from the day she was born.

One memory I hold deep in my heart is standing on my desk when my father came to my school to share the news Andrea was born and cheering that the baby was a girl. My twin brother Paul wasn't quite as excited with the news! Little did I know that God had dropped her from heaven to be my forever loving sister who lets me be my true self and who I know will be by my side no matter what.

The moment Andrea picked up the phone, I trembled, whispering, "Taylor has cancer." According to Andrea, I didn't say, "might have," and I'm not sure why. Although Taylor's diagnosis hadn't yet officially been confirmed and although I too pleaded with God for this to be one big mistake, in my heart of hearts I somehow knew the truth. Andrea too was so shaken by this news that she completely forgot to feed Samantha, her then-fifteen-month-old baby, all day and wondered why she refused to settle. Samantha's cries of hunger may've been frenzied, but they were no match for Andrea's. Suddenly I saw Bob and blurted out, "Andrea, I have to go!"

After the CT scan, Bob, Taylor, and I were placed in a waiting room in the pediatric oncology suite or, as I saw it, a holding pen awaiting our death sentence. Taylor did her best to amuse herself, oblivious to the other kids playing in the waiting room. She seemed not to notice that most of them were bald, some missing limbs or bandaged from surgery. Several were pushing IV poles tethered to their arms. In fact, she wasn't overly concerned about anything other than getting food.

When the doctor finally summoned us, she averted her eyes. We followed her, single file, like three little ducks. She sat us down in her sterile office and asked, "Taylor, can you hop on the exam table?" As Taylor walked across the room, I watched her every step, one moment thinking I could see her cancer, the next thinking, *See how well she walks? She doesn't have cancer!* At the same time, I was frozen and trapped in time, not hearing, seeing, or feeling much of anything. The doctor, whose face and name escape me but whose squeaky, hollow voice I will never forget, asked Taylor to perform the standard tests one would have at an annual checkup: "Taylor, squeeze my hand; let me look at your spine." She then asked Taylor to leave the room, and somehow, I allowed it. I still berate myself for letting her leave and sit outside all alone.

The doctor mercifully opted for the direct but sensitive approach. She smiled in that "I'm so sorry" kind of way and in a serious tone confirmed what I already knew: "Your child has cancer. It appears to be bone cancer, and yet it seems to have started in the neural tissue. We can't be sure yet. She will need to be admitted to the hospital right away for tests."

We knew that admission into the hospital was possible but hearing it jolted us. I asked the only question I knew to ask about cancer: "What stage is she?" The doctor shook her head and explained that this type of pediatric cancer wasn't normally "staged" the way we were used to thinking. She looked back at us as she paused, swallowed, and finally said, "In those kind of terms, she is stage four." Those shocking, ugly words engulfed me like a tidal wave. How could this be? Taylor had been in school that very morning.

I found myself wanting to rewind the clock to just one night prior, when I had happily tucked each of my three girls into bed and slept peacefully myself. That was the last day of "before," and I had no idea what the journey of "after" would entail.

A Weighty Task

Bob and I had a brief discussion about what to do next: I would head home to somehow tell our daughters their sister had cancer and pack a bag for a hospital stay of unknown length. As unimaginable as that seemed to me, I didn't envy Bob his task. He had to tell Taylor.

After I left, the two of them sat on a bench outside the pediatric oncology waiting room, staring into space and waiting to be admitted. Taylor knew she needed to stay in the hospital for tests, but in all our shock, we hadn't told Tales why. She slipped her hand in Bob's, and he almost started crying right there. She looked up at him and asked, "Daddy, why do I have to stay in the hospital?"

Bob could feel his face flush and wondered if she could see it. You make some of the most important decisions in your life in the split second it takes to process a question. He decided right there that he would never lie to Taylor, and though we didn't always tell her everything we knew, we never were dishonest. Gingerly, he murmured, "Tales, the doctors think you have cancer, and they need to do some tests." She didn't answer but snuggled against Bob, beginning to get teary. Then Taylor looked at him again, searching his face as she cried, and asked, "Am I going to die?"

The first question left him breathless, but this one left him hollowed out. He thought, *How can I be holding my little eleven-year-old daughter and be answering this question?* With grace and strength, he answered, "Tales, we all have to die sometime, but this is not your time." She looked at him for a few seconds, seemed satisfied, and never, ever, asked the question again.

As Taylor was drying her eyes, the oncologist walked by and paused, noticing Taylor's tears. She raised her eyebrows and looked puzzled.

"Taylor, you look upset."

Taylor nodded.

"Taylor, you know this is what I do for a living, right? I have seen this problem many, many times. I know exactly what to do."

At that moment, she was practicing medicine at its best. Taylor looked at her, and back at Bob, and smiled. She sat up, and she wiped her eyes in the defiant way she had done her whole life.

The doctor smiled. "We'll see each other tomorrow, okay?"

And with that, Taylor waved, the doctor waved, and the battle began.

The next question from Taylor was classic: "Daddy, is chemo the medicine that makes cancer people get skinny and look so weak?"

"Yes, sweetie, chemo can make it very hard to keep up your weight and your strength," Bob responded. She hesitated for a moment to read Bob's face, then exclaimed, "Daddy, let's go out for pizza!" At this point, she was allowed to eat, as we were told she wouldn't be having another scan that day. Taylor always had a voracious appetite, but nothing could prepare Bob to watch her eat almost an entire large pizza by herself. Knowing he was headed back to the hospital, he chuckled, thinking maybe they'd have to stop by the emergency room for a stomach pump.

Meanwhile, I had the job of telling the rest of our family, starting with my parents. I couldn't help but remember our conversation right after Taylor was born. My dad, whose voice and accent sound like a combination of Bernie Sanders and Fred Flintstone, answered, "Hullo?" and then in a booming voice, "What? What did you name her, Susan?" I laughed. Everyone in my life calls me "Sue," but he refuses to call me anything but "Susan." He went on. "What kind of name is Taylor Anne? You mean like the stores, Lord and Taylor, or Ann Taylor?" I smiled. "Yes, Daddy."

I dialed the phone.

"Hello?"

"Hi, Mom, it's me. Can you put Daddy on the phone?" My voice was thick and guttural, sounding like it was coming from someone else. Uncharacteristically, my mother didn't ask any questions but instead put my father on the phone immediately.

"Daddy," I whispered, "Taylor has cancer." And then, as with all children young or old, the sound of my father's voice gave me the freedom to let out the first of many more cries and screams to come. "Help me, Daddy!" I shouted. I don't remember how he responded, but I know he was in sheer disbelief.

My mother, physically petite but emotionally charged, grabbed the phone, and yelled, "Taylor does *not* have cancer." Rita was a piece of work; she had a huge personality, talked incessantly to anyone within earshot, and argued about absolutely everything for sport. Before call waiting, sometimes Andrea would be on the phone with her and they'd somehow get disconnected. Andrea would try calling back for the longest time and keep getting a busy signal, because Rita didn't realize Andrea wasn't on the other end for all that time. She just continued talking—to herself!

Rita insisted, "Taylor was here last night taking a piano lesson, and she was fine. There's been a mistake. She doesn't look sick, and if she were, we'd know it. Believe me." It would take my mom several months to admit Taylor had cancer.

Her reaction was not surprising. She didn't believe in doctors and, therefore, never went to them. She died at seventy-four after only having one mammogram. My mom's response to medical situations was to ignore them, justifying her decisions by telling us, "All doctors want is to find something wrong with you to make money." This was precisely the reason I always brought my children to the doctor immediately when something was wrong and why I insisted on seeing a pulmonologist when all we thought Taylor had was exercise-induced asthma: when it came to doctors, I did the polar opposite of what my mom did.

When I arrived home, I walked inside and immediately hugged Dotsie, our trusted eighty-year-old babysitter. Dotsie—the name Ryan bestowed on her when she couldn't pronounce her real name, Dorothy—had been caring for my girls for thirteen years. Corey was nestled in Dotsie's lap as they read a book—she was a little snuggle-bunny. Corey was very precocious, loved school and her friends, and was a happy, carefree eight-year-old with a voracious appetite for learning. As the youngest of three girls, she freely borrowed her sisters' clothes and decked herself out. She certainly did not dress or, in some ways, act like an average third grader. I remembered one time, a year or so prior, when she questioned our tour guide about his facts and ended up being correct! When we asked how she knew those facts, she rattled off even more details, telling us, "It was in a book I read." *Really? At age seven?*

"Corey, Mommy needs to talk to you about something important."

"What, Mommy?" she said in her innocent, high-pitched voice.

"The doctors told us today that Taylor is sick, that she has something called cancer. She's going to be okay, but we are going to have to give her a lot of medicine for the next few months to make her better."

Corey's face became pale with concern. "Oh, no, Mommy, but where is she?"

"She's at the hospital, sweetheart, and Mommy has to go back there soon and stay with her tonight. Daddy will be home with you and Ryan though, so don't worry."

A tear rolled slowly down her cheek. "But, Mommy, I lost a tooth today. Does this mean that the tooth fairy won't come tonight?"

I embraced her, letting myself experience what life had been just yesterday.

"Of course the tooth fairy will come, sweetheart." Our family tradition was to give the girls a nickel, a penny, and a dollar amount that corresponded to the number of teeth they had lost. That night I had no time or cognitive ability to count how many teeth Corey had lost, so I gave Dotsie a twenty-dollar bill, only later finding out that breaking tradition would clue Corey in and rob her of believing a little fairy, who always knew exactly how many teeth she had lost, flew into her room at night to exchange her tooth for money.

Telling our older daughter Ryan, an eighth grader, was grueling. I left Corey with Dotsie and went to pick Ryan up from lacrosse practice at the high school. As I approached the coach to ask for Ryan's release, I blurted out the news to several parents standing by. I moved through the crowd as if in slow motion, every step heavy and deliberate, until I reached my daughter, who looked concerned. As we left the field together, I embraced Ryan and in a barely audible tone whispered, "Taylor has cancer." She stared at me and began to cry, shoulders shaking. Neither of us remembers what we said next, but I will never forget her face, contorted in agony and fear, covered in black mascara-stained tears.

Ryan and I rushed home to pack a bag for Taylor. Almost as soon as I had arrived, I had to leave. When I had a moment alone, I stared at the floor, clutching my thighs and breathing deeply, trying to maintain composure and muster the courage to leave my girls after telling them the worst news of their lives. It was an agonizing but unavoidable choice, one that I would unfortunately have to make countless times in the years to come. The tooth fairy was only the first casualty.

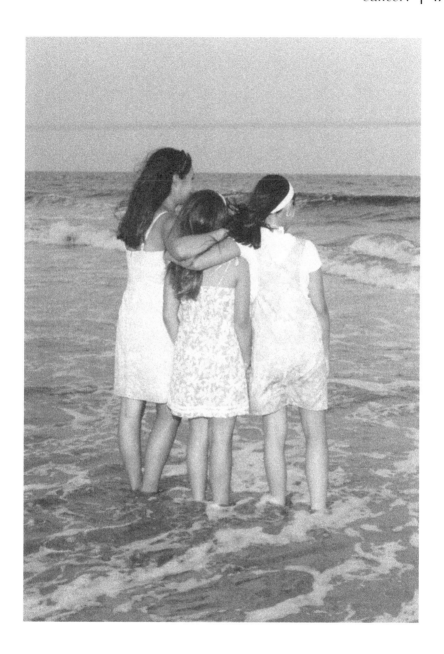

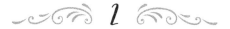

A Rude Awakening

Love is the emblem of eternity: it confounds all notion of time: it effaces all memory of a beginning, all fear of an end.

–Anne Louise Germaine De Stael

Stark-White Reality

By the time I returned to the hospital, Taylor was already hooked up to an IV pole. The room looked stark, white, and sterile, as any hospital room would be. Yet it took me by surprise. What was I thinking—that it would be a plush, brightly colored, happy place? I needed Taylor to be back in her cheery yellow and blue room filled with all the things she loved: her glow-in-the-dark clock, her favorite stuffed animals Bun-Bun and Oatmeal, and her desk overflowing with the pictures and quirky knick-knacks she had gathered over the years. Just last night she had been on the phone, nestled under her blankets, secretly speaking to her sixth-grade "boyfriend" Warnell.

Late that night, Andrea called back. Taylor said in a sheepish tone, without sounding particularly worried, "They say I have cancer."

"I heard, Tales. But don't worry. Cancer used to be a bad thing, but today it isn't. They'll be able to treat you, no problem."

"Yeah," Taylor replied. Perking up, she added, "And now I get to eat all the candy I want!"

Andrea smiled, thinking, *Of course that's how Tales would see it.*

Taylor finally fell asleep as I sat beside her. All day long I had felt frozen and trapped in time, not hearing, seeing, or feeling much of anything, unable to process what was happening. Emotionally, I was in the eye of a hurricane, and though it was quiet and dark in that moment, I recognized it for what it was: peace before chaos. And that's when the tears let loose.

I lay in that dark hospital room and silently wept deep into the night, my eyes swollen, red, and sore as I blew my nose and soaked up the constant flow of tears with my shirt. Any sense of dignity was already gone. At the same time, I couldn't stop looking at my sweet and innocent baby, making sure she was still breathing. She seemed to be peacefully sleeping while holding on to my hand. I knew she wouldn't notice if I let go, but I didn't dare. She was my anchor, keeping me steady that night and, indeed, forevermore.

My sadness transformed into all-encompassing fear when, at two o'clock in the morning, the nurse startled us by barging in: "Taylor needs a CT scan of her brain." Taylor didn't seem alarmed, but how could she not be? The night before, she was warm and snug in her bed, without a care in the world. Twenty-four hours later, she was on a hospital gurney getting a brain scan.

When they wheeled Taylor into the scan room and shut the door in my face, I slid down the wall and hit the hard, frigid floor, where I cried and screamed, hoping and praying the cancer had not spread to Taylor's brain. I kept telling myself not to worry. She was the same Taylor: bright, feisty, and fun. Nothing about her, other than her diagnosis, seemed to have changed.

The following morning, hours felt like minutes as we wandered around like zombies. The brain scan was clear, but we knew things were, nevertheless, bad, based on the forced smiles and artificial cheeriness emanating from the nurses. The most concerned among the physicians was the surgeon, who explained that Taylor needed a biopsy of her tumor to identify the type of cancer she had. He said without pause, "The procedure is challenging, dangerous, and possibly life threatening."

Without thinking, I snapped, "My daughter was in school yesterday, and today you're telling me she's having a procedure that could be life threatening? Just tell me this: who is taking the IV out, you or me? Because we are getting the hell out of here!" Making rash decisions in times of crisis can be a mistake, but in this moment, I instinctively knew we had to run far and fast to get out of our local hospital and over to a major cancer institution. A family friend, who was a physician, facilitated an immediate admission into Memorial Sloan Kettering Cancer Center in New York City, known as one of the premiere cancer centers in the world.

I am not sure how any parent initially chooses the hospital in which to treat his or her child. The urgency and shock of diagnosis is so severe one's mind can't focus, and most parents don't question a thing. In our frenzy, we picked the hospital with the best reputation, without researching other institutions or the actual doctors who would be treating Taylor. We had no idea of how anything in the medical world worked.

Before we could leave the hospital and head to Sloan, a nurse came to find me. I was sitting in a dim corridor amongst a pile of IV poles. She asked for my insurance card. I blankly asked, "Why?" somehow irrationally fearing that giving her our insurance card would prevent us from leaving. The nurse politely responded, "Taylor cannot leave the hospital without medical transport." I handed over my card, and we waited for as long as we could for an ambulance, eventually deciding we would drive her ourselves. An understanding nurse removed her IV, and we walked out of the hospital. How were we to know that this is strictly forbidden by hospital protocol? Day one, and we had already broken the rules!

Once at Sloan we waited in a plush room filled with toys, children's artwork, and comfortable, cozy chairs. A smiling nurse greeted us, as any concierge would, welcoming us to Taylor's hotel, aka hospital room, which became almost immediately a party room. Several nurses greeted Taylor with brand new toys and made her laugh.

Taylor looked so good walking around, sporting a white shirt and light pink pants, the hospital staff mistook her for a sibling rather than the cancer patient. Her file, of course, described a critically sick kid. Yet we breathed a sigh of relief and, like most desperate parents, hung on to every word the doctors said, assigning meaning to even the slightest nod or smile. As if because the doctor thinks she's a sibling, she must not have cancer. What a joke! Later we would find out that due to the extent of cancer in Taylor's lungs, the doctors had assumed she wouldn't be able to walk.

We barely got our feet on the ground before we were bombarded with treatment plans, biopsy results, scan dates, and words we could not pronounce, let alone understand. As I was trying to make sense of this new world into which I was suddenly thrust, my intuition again reminded me that my most important job was to maintain my composure so as to not scare Taylor. I kept silently repeating to myself, *No matter what, she has to believe that Mommy and Daddy will make everything all better.* In this regard, my instincts were spot on.

Meanwhile, word of Taylor's diagnosis moved quickly throughout our community. We weren't able to answer calls or emails, texting didn't yet exist, and we couldn't bear to repeatedly tell the story. Within a day of diagnosis, Bob somehow had the wherewithal to start an online journal. Eloquently, and with great compassion and humor, he relayed Taylor's story. Many of his journal entries were written in the middle of the night. They were honest and accurate but rarely told details of the trauma we were experiencing, because sometimes Taylor and her friends read it, and we didn't want anything to interfere with her optimism and drive.

Aside from the urgency of dealing with Taylor's diagnosis, we had to find someone immediately to help us with Ryan and Corey. Dotsie didn't believe a child could have cancer, let alone Taylor. She was in total denial and not functioning at all. I knew within two days that Dotsie would not be able to handle watching my girls on a full-time basis, and my parents and siblings were unable or unwilling to help. My mom's own illness had just started to take hold, and my father was caring for her; my brother worked full-time, and Andrea lived in North Carolina. Lynn, who lived fifteen minutes away, was clearly not going to help. In a later conversation, she told me, "I can't come because it hurts my children too much to see Taylor."

What was I to do? This full-time mom suddenly needed to find a substitute, under the worst possible conditions and at a moment's notice. During the first few days after diagnosis, I had no idea what was going on at home with my other children. Ryan has since told me, "I'll never forget walking into the drab but normal school hallway, totally numb, confused, and not sure what was happening in the hospital with my sister." The second she walked through the door, people with pitying eyes inundated her with questions. "It was like being caught naked when you thought you were alone," she said. "My heart raced; I didn't know that everyone knew, and I didn't have any answers to their questions, nor was I ready to talk about it."

I knew I was not going to be able to be present for my other girls physically or emotionally; I didn't trust myself. From Sloan, in a state of total confusion, I interviewed several "sitters" but had no idea what questions to ask, not knowing what I even needed, with no time to figure it out. We ended up settling on a part-time sitter for the summer, whom we found through the grace of a friend's recommendation.

Come fall, the search intensified until we met the ultimate solution through a friend of a friend: Beata. Call it a mother's intuition, but I knew immediately that she would love my girls, treat them as if they were her own, and grasp the gravity of the situation. With her long, cascading honey-blonde curls, her Polish accent, and enthusiasm for life, she nurtured and fed my children's souls. It felt like a miracle.

The Infamous Éclair

Five days after Taylor was diagnosed, she needed surgery to insert a Broviac. Of course, we had no idea what that was, but we soon learned a Broviac is an intravenous catheter channeled under the skin, eventually reaching a large vein that goes directly to the heart. The soft, white tubes at the end of the catheter exit the body, allowing chemotherapy to be given through the tubes, thus completely avoiding the need for an IV. Most cancer patients are given either a Broviac or a port, a similar device surgically placed under one's skin.

Right after surgery, with alarming eyes, Taylor blurted, "Mommy! I feel a weird flutter in my heart." I called the nurse immediately. She changed Taylor's position in bed, which stopped the fluttering, and we didn't think too much more about it.

The following morning, I asked Taylor what she wanted for breakfast, even though I knew the answer: "An éclair, Mommy!" When I gave it to her, she smiled brightly and devoured her very favorite food. That would be the last éclair she ever ate.

Suddenly, Taylor's heart monitors shrieked, jolting me like a bolt of lightning. Every flash of red and clamorous beep felt like a hammer on my head. I became completely hysterical. I had no idea what was wrong.

Within five minutes, two surgeons dressed in vibrant yellow surgical gowns were bedside. The Broviac catheter had entered Taylor's heart, causing a dire situation. It needed to be surgically repositioned immediately. However, because she had eaten the now-infamous éclair, she could not have general anesthesia. The situation was too grave to wait. The doctors literally started cutting Taylor open bedside with just a local anesthetic, while Bob held her hand steadily and calmly.

As I watched my daughter's red blood spouting everywhere and the terror in her eyes, anger gripped my neck, threatening to suffocate me. This was human error! The Broviac obviously was inserted incorrectly, and as soon as we told the nurse about the fluttering in Taylor's heart, she should have contacted the surgeon. I wanted to leap on the nurse's back and kick and scream, "My sweet, innocent child, who was playing like any other child on the playground last week, now has to go through this barbaric procedure because of you!"

Later, I was speaking to Taylor's nurse practitioner, Karen, a heavy-set woman whose ox-like demeanor initially had scared us until we got to know her warm side. She told me, "Sue, I couldn't introduce myself or comfort you during that awful Broviac fiasco because you were curled up in a ball, in the fetal position, out of sight of the surgery." I was astounded and completely baffled. According to her, I didn't personally witness the surgery. I understand that sometimes my memories are hazy. However, this memory is remarkably vivid. How could it contain fallacies? On the other hand, Bob remembers I wasn't on the floor in the fetal position but sitting in a chair, disengaged, watching from a distance. Either way, I could swear I was right there next to Taylor while this was happening.

Afterwards, Taylor, with folded arms, remarked accusingly, "Daddy held me tight. He wasn't crying. He told me I would be okay, and he didn't scare me." He held her hand for dear life and protected his baby girl the best he could, while I, without even fully realizing it, apparently went someplace far, far away, somewhere over the rainbow.

From that moment on, throughout Taylor's illness, Bob and I each took on certain roles and responsibilities: Bob alone would meet with the doctors, while I stayed with Taylor. I was responsible for Taylor's day-to-day care: tracking all of her medications, learning how to minimize her suffering, and making chemo life fun. Bob, on the other hand, diligently researched treatments online almost every night and got many second, third, fourth, and fifth opinions. This strategy worked well for us, as Taylor never felt abandoned and I didn't have to hear what the doctors had to say. Bob was the strong one. We never stopped being a team and worked extremely hard to complement each other throughout her battle.

Taylor knew Bob studied, read, and called hospitals and doctors all over the world. He listened to the doctors' news and then formed meaningful questions in response. Over time he learned he had to question them at every turn and demand more information than they were usually willing to give. It was anything but easy, yet he never let up. She knew he made a pot of coffee every night after she went to bed and stayed up half the night reading research papers and studying results so that he could create lists of alternatives to ask the doctors about.

Each night, Tales would ask her daddy, "What is next?" and he would tell her what he thought. I would often find them totally immersed in conversation. She trusted him to make the decisions more than she trusted her doctors, and she always believed there was a next step. She would listen intently, absorbing all of the science and the vocabulary, and then, at some point, peacefully close her eyes, ready for sleep.

Bob's fierce diligence, tenacity, and refusal to give up saved Tales many times over and gave her the hope to continue battling. He is the true hero of Taylor's journey. They were quite a pair. I was greatly comforted knowing that the job of being our family's advocate was in his ever-so-capable and tireless hands. He worked all day, researched all night, and never complained.

A Bad Hair Day

About a week into diagnosis, listening to the sound of running water while Taylor was in the hospital shower, I silently sobbed. I knew it would be one of the last times, for a long time, she would feel the suds cascading down her long chestnut-brown hair. Gleaming and satiny, her hair was the kind I loved to run my hands through. I wondered if Taylor had yet connected the dots and realized it would soon fall out.

I shivered as I heard the clanking of the rusty faucet turning off, quickly wiped my tears, and thought about the person Taylor was inside. Was I the only one anxious about this? She was beautiful but never vain. I used to beg her to shop for clothes, but all she ever wanted to wear were the same pair of ugly, comfortable, elastic-waist pants in every color from the Gap. "Who cares what I look like, Mommy?" she would argue. Maybe Taylor would be okay with the dreaded words a mother never dares to think she will have to tell her daughter.

When my angel came out of the shower wrapped in two towels, one on her head and one on her body, I gestured for her to come cuddle on my lap. As I caressed her face, I gently explained, "Tales, within two weeks, you are going to lose your hair." She didn't say a word, tightened her grip around my shoulders, and breathed deeply, taking the air from my lungs directly into hers. A few tears silently slipped down her porcelain face, wetting my sleeve. She peacefully rested her head on my shoulder. The moment was so tender. We held each other for as long as I can remember, and although the circumstances were dire, it is those times that I cherish the most—the moments of sheer unconditional love shared between mother and child.

As her wet towel and soft tears dampened my shirt and shattered my heart, Taylor taught me the first of many life lessons. No one would wish cancer on his or her worst enemy, but there can be some good that comes out of it. If you let it, cancer slows life down just long enough to afford you opportunities to hold close the ones you love, breathe in their scent, feel their skin upon yours, and unwaveringly thank God for bringing them into your life. As long as we had each other, nothing else mattered.

In that moment, I was reminded of one of the kids' favorite Dr. Seuss Christmas movies: "And what happened, then? Well, in Whoville they say that the Grinch's small heart grew three sizes that day." Trapped within the four walls of a cold, dank, and alien hospital room, where fear tried its best to strangle me and convert all my love to anger, instead my heart grew bigger. Cancer changed a lot, but it can't change that.

Two days before Taylor's sixth-grade graduation party, a party that I had been planning all year with the other PTA moms, clumps of her locks fell out. I panicked, as there was no missing this party. She had already missed her actual graduation ceremony because it was a chemo day. Her school principal, Dr. Kennedy, whose kindness and understanding is only matched by his intellect, had asked me with great compassion, "Can you reschedule chemo and let her attend graduation?" I had adamantly declined, explaining, "Postponing treatment would be impossible."

I wish I had known then what I know now, but it was all part of the learning curve. We quickly realized that a successful cancer journey is all about *living* life while in treatment. You can't put your entire life on hold and watch it pass before your eyes. The only way to get through treatment is to have fun whenever you possibly can. From that point forward, Taylor, Bob, and I fought the medical system and began doing things our way. Taylor was never again going to miss an important event.

Taylor, who like all adolescents wanted nothing more than to fit in, was overcome with worry. She wailed, "Mommy! Why can't I have my hair for another two days?" I had no answer as my stomach dropped and my heart sank. Taylor needed to wear a bandana for her graduation party.

I conveyed my concern to one of Taylor's close friend's mom. Without hesitation, she said. "Don't worry, Sue; we will make this okay for Taylor." On a moment's notice, she purchased bandanas for all the girls to wear so that Taylor would feel more comfortable at the party. The girls felt grown up, as they were about to enter junior high, and were ready to show it. But in support of Taylor, they ditched their flat irons and donned brightly colored bandanas. Taylor felt normal that night, a true blessing.

A few days later, Taylor asked with a rueful laugh, "Daddy, can you shave my head? It's so itchy." It is a moment I'll never forget; it played out in screaming color against a gray backdrop that had suddenly and unapologetically become our new world. Taylor had already cut her long, straight hair into short layers, a hairstyle any eleven-year-old would never consider. She did it for entertainment value, knowing she would soon be bald.

Bob and I were astounded and wildly humbled at how she could find humor in this situation. Just that week, Bob had come home, saying, "I bought the kit to shave my head, too." Taylor had laughed and said, "Great, Daddy, we will both be bald." We just didn't think it would be so soon.

As he shaved away his beautiful daughter's hair, Bob's soul was torn apart, piece-by-piece. The pain in his heart and the courage it took for him to run the electric razor and then the Gillette razor up and down with a steady hand was never betrayed by his smile. He fought with every ounce of his being to keep Taylor from being afraid. I trembled, unable to hold back my tears, but Taylor didn't shed one.

After Bob finished shaving her head, he bravely offered, without a hint of regret, "Okay, Tales; it's my turn!" Taylor surprised us both and adamantly said, "No, Daddy! I don't want you to do it." She would never tell us why she changed her mind.

Her sisters were downstairs and had no idea any of this was going on. It was a special day, Corey's ninth birthday. I am sure Taylor did not plan to shave her head on Corey's birthday, but to this day, it bothers me. After Tales was cleaned up, she ran down the stairs, struck a pose as if modeling for a fashion show, and boasted, "Look at me!" I peeked into the room through our glass French doors, watching their interactions. I imagine her sisters were terrified, but they didn't show a sign of it. They always had her back. Both girls hugged Taylor and laughed right alongside her, as if she had merely shared a funny joke. No words were spoken. As horrific as the situation was, the love shared between my three daughters was abounding.

Only later Ryan told me, "Mommy, I was so scared. Seeing Taylor bald made everything so much more real." Corey's recollection of seeing Taylor newly bald, on the other hand, speaks volumes. She doesn't recall any of it.

Years later we received a call from a mother with a newly diagnosed little girl. She asked, "What should I do?" Taylor quickly replied, "Tell her to dye her hair pink or a combination of all her favorite colors." She would later tell others, "If you are a boy, cut it into a Mohawk; try layers and new styles; get bangs. Be outrageous!" In retrospect, before shaving it off, we should have painted Taylor's hair blue, her favorite color.

A Worthy Cause

The shock of diagnosis soon gave way to the alarming reality that treatments for Taylor's particular disease had not changed in decades. Can you imagine telling your eleven-year-old child this information? Taylor was aghast: "How do kids like me get cancer treatments that are as old as you and Daddy?" We laughed, trying to hide the ominous truth. Unless you are in the world of pediatric cancer, this is a well-guarded secret. What enraged Taylor and fueled us was that the United States government provides little funding for childhood cancer research. All childhood cancers combined receive only approximately 4 percent of the National Cancer Institute's budget.

Taylor put her feelings into her own words:

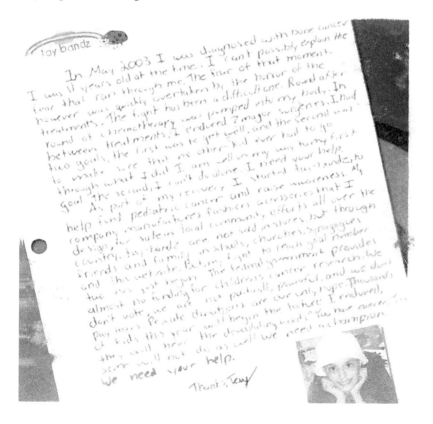

To win the battle, you have to know the basic facts (see cac2.org):

- Cancer is the number one cause of death by disease among children in the United States.
- The average five-year survival rate when considered as a whole is 83 percent. Therefore, approximately one in five children diagnosed with cancer will die in the first five years.
- One in 285 children will be diagnosed with cancer before the age of twenty.
- Approximately 35 percent of children diagnosed with cancer will die within thirty years of diagnosis.
- Those who survive the five years have an eight times greater mortality rate.
- More than 95 percent of childhood cancer survivors will have a significant health-related issue by the time they are forty-five years old; these health-related issues are side effects of either the cancer or, more commonly, the result of its treatment. One-third will suffer chronic side effects; one-third will suffer moderate to severe health problems, and one-third will have severe or life-threatening conditions.

Despite these facts, the issues surrounding childhood cancer are consistently misunderstood. Taylor was horrified that thousands of children could be suffering from cancer, yet their cries for help were being ignored. Taylor was determined to make a difference. Less than a month after diagnosis, she founded a grassroots nonprofit 501(c)(3) organization in our local community whose sole mission is to raise awareness and fund pediatric cancer research. Taylor aptly named it "tay-bandz," for her nickname Tay and for headbands, the first product made. She dreamed that "someday, no child would ever have to face cancer," and repeatedly told me, "Mommy, if I could save the life of one child, it would all be worth it."

Taylor, being only eleven years old, thought the best way to fundraise was to sell goods, but she decided she did not want tay-bandz to simply be an arts-and-crafts project. She wanted to sell products that were professionally made. Big dreams aside, when she first started tay-bandz, none of us had any idea the money raised would ever become something other than the equivalent of a large school bake sale.

The launch of her business was the brainchild of our friend, Jill, and our neighbors who had professional experience in retail. They helped Taylor source the materials and had them manufactured to Taylor's specifications. Taylor designed her logo one summer night at dinner while coloring on a napkin. She asked, "Do you think I should include a rainbow and a ladybug?" two of her favorite symbols of life and luck. Bob replied, "Of course, Tales; this is your project." She lifted her head, put down the paper, and smiled the type of smile that melts your heart. She was just a kid with aspirations and a box of crayons.

At one point, Taylor was well enough to go on an adventure to pick out fabric and ribbons herself. We set out for New York City's garment district, a section of the city that measures about one square mile, also known as the "fashion mecca." Taylor carefully selected rolls of ribbon and fabric, amazed at how many choices she had. She exploded with excitement, the wheels in her brain spinning with ideas for future products.

As we were leaving one of the stores, I said, "Shoot, it's pouring outside. Stay here; I will get the car." I could barely get the words out before Tales raced out the door, jumping up and down with her arms held open wide. She was literally dancing in the rain! I joined her, and she exclaimed, "Mommy, I haven't felt rain since I got sick. It feels awesome on my bald head!" I was stunned, never expecting Taylor's response to the rain, while kicking myself for not realizing how much we had taken for granted prior to her illness.

Taylor's foundation, tay-bandz, helped Taylor through her own cancer journey. In an interview on CBS, she said, "When I was sad, sick, missing my sisters and my friends, I knew I should go and design, because I would be helping the people after me who didn't feel well. Knowing they may be getting treatments that I funded research for is really great." Taylor was astounded when she raised her first $100,000. She knew we were thrilled, but I don't think she truly understood until she was older what all those zeros meant.

A Moment That Makes Life Worthwhile

As treatment continued, Taylor persevered with strength, fortitude, and a glass-half-full attitude. But chemo is not for the faint of heart. Soon Taylor's suffering became agonizing, with no end in sight. What more could they do to her? Never ask that question.

One evening, I came into our bathroom at home to prepare Tales for a shower. Her Broviac tubes needed to be completely covered in plastic wrap, like a cast would. I found her gazing into the mirror. Her skin was a putrid shade of green, she was completely bald with no eyebrows or eyelashes, and tubes were jutting out of her body. She was bone thin. She must have been looking at herself in horror. Anyone would be frightened. How could an eleven-year-old possibly make sense of what cancer had done to her body?

My head reeled at the pain she was experiencing both physically and mentally. Yet although her outer beauty had dissipated, her inner beauty remained intact. As I entered the room, she smiled brightly, not wanting me to see her despair. Neither of us said a word. She got into the shower as sadness pierced my soul. As I slumped on the bathroom floor, she cleared the mist from the shower door, saw me, and wrote, "I ♥ you." I believe she wanted me to know that love overcomes everything.

Now, when I take a shower, I often draw a heart and many times a droplet of water drips down, cutting the heart in half. Although my heart breaks a little bit more with each passing day, my love affair with my daughter continues to bloom brighter and bigger. We don't measure Taylor's life in sunrises; we measure her life in love.

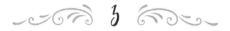

Think Outside the Box

The chief conditions on which life, health and vigor depend on is action.

–Colin Powell

Fluffy Friends

Let me start by saying I was never a pet person until our boxer became part of our family. I grew up with a miniature dachshund named Binky, but he was much more Lynn's dog than he was mine. After I moved out, two more dachshunds would eventually move into my childhood home and become part of the family. Andrea's dog was Pesto, whom she worshipped, constantly singing to him in a childlike voice and carrying on ridiculously about how much she loved him. When I was putting together a fortieth birthday album for Andrea with pictures from her life, apparently I put in a picture of Pesto and jotted on the side of the book, "What's this dog's name? I can't remember."

"Sue!" she shrieked upon seeing the entry. "How could you not recognize Pesto? What is wrong with you?" It was as if I couldn't remember the name of one of her kids, she was so appalled, but really, it's just not my thing, never was.

Anyone who has kids knows most badger their parents to get a pet. My kids excelled at that! Bob and I eventually gave in and bought a rambunctious boxer whom we named "Socks" for her white paws. She joined the family as the fifth female. Poor Bob! She was a sweet, tender, and loving boxer with a grand personality who could knock anyone over with her exuberance. Believe it or not, I did really love this dog.

Fabulous as Socks was, within the first weeks after Taylor was diagnosed, she begged for another dog, desperately wanting someone new with whom to cuddle. Socks was anything but a cuddly puffball. Here we go again, puppy poop and crate training. We couldn't say no to Taylor, and the little devil knew it.

After much research, Taylor chose a Cavalier King Charles Spaniel. Taylor asked her dear friend Laura to come with us to pick him out. Laura and Taylor had a very special relationship. Somehow, they had named each other "Butthead," with Laura being "Butt" and Taylor being "Head," and that was how it stayed. Together we trekked out to Long Island to speak with the breeder, an elderly woman whose home smelled of dog pee. She took one look at Taylor and instantly told her, "You can pick the puppy of your choice." To our surprise, she chose a male dog. This puppy would be the first-ever male in the family besides Bob. Taylor named him Lucky. He was eleven weeks old, was tricolored with black, white, and patches of gold around his face, and had big, brown, button eyes. He was adorable, but time would tell if Lucky's fate matched his name.

Shortly after we brought Lucky home, I was in the hospital with Taylor, engaged in conversation with her doctors, when my phone began ringing repeatedly. I finally retrieved it and heard Corey's voice, somewhere between screaming and crying. She was nine at the time. "Mommy, when Lucky, this stupid dog Taylor wanted, plays with my stuffed animals, he gets on top of them, and this long pointy thing comes out of his wiener. Thennnnnn, my favorite pink FAO Schwartz dog got covered in all this gook. My stuffed animal is ruined!" Taylor could see me desperately trying to hold back laughter while simultaneously attempting to calm Corey down. She grabbed the phone out of my hand and said, "Enough, Cor. He is just having fun."

Neutering Lucky unfortunately did nothing to help. After several more male-centered debacles, the family agreed it was time for Lucky to go. Bob learned an important family lesson. Act too male, and you might be excommunicated! We gave him to a person dear to us. It was an easy decision for everyone, except for poor Lucky, the sexually promiscuous spaniel.

One evening, I walked into Taylor's hospital room to find her hanging out with one of her favorite nurses, Julie, who was sporting pigtails. She had classic curly hair, the type no straightener could every touch. She placed one of her pigtails over Taylor's bald head, making Tales look like a puppy. I laughed, watching my daughter pretend to be a dog as if she was three years old. Next thing I knew, she had her sights on a new breed.

This time Tales decided she wanted a Mi-Ki, a rare toy breed that almost no one had heard of. There were only two Mi-Ki breeders in the United States at the time. Taylor contacted both of them but was disappointed to learn the next few litters were already promised to other customers. Always unstoppable, somehow Taylor convinced one of the breeders to give her a female dog within a few weeks. Mi-Kis are smooth and long-coated with large brown eyes, apparently seldom bark, and have lively and friendly dispositions. The breed seemed a good fit for our family. But although I knew Taylor wanted a cuddly, small dog, I believe the real reason she chose a Mi-Ki was because its history is shrouded in secrecy. The myths and legends continue to propagate. Even today, the combination of breeds resulting in a Mi-Ki is still uncertain. The more intrigue and mystery in Taylor's life, the happier she was.

The next thing I knew, we were driving to Newark Airport to pick up our Mi-Ki, who was flying up from Florida. We all decided to name her Jessie. Without an immune system, Taylor could not enter the airport. While double-parked outside the United Airlines terminal, I swiftly ran inside, identified the flight attendant who had agreed to provide transport, and peeked into the tiny crate. With dozens of thank-yous, I scooted off, holding one very precious little pup. The exchange took less than five minutes.

Taylor gingerly held Jessie in the palm of her hand for the entire ride home. Her joy was a ray of sunshine, but it didn't last. Jessie was an adorable, snow-colored little puffball, but she had little personality and barked in a squeaky and annoying voice. In retrospect, maybe we didn't give Jessie a fair chance, because Socks had such a vibrant personality. However, she was a keeper, particularly because she was female and a great playmate for Socks. Each evening, Jessie fell asleep spooning with Socks. It was their love story.

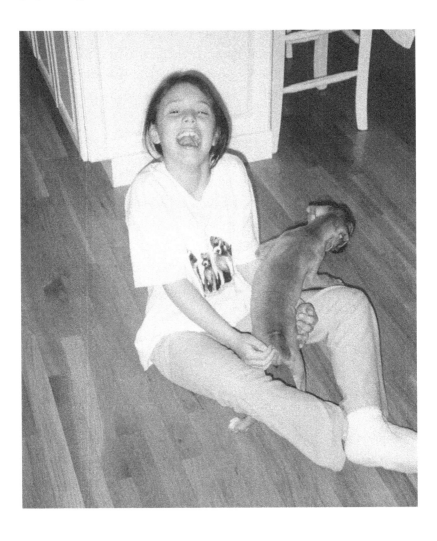

My Heart Will Go On

A month later, in August 2003, Taylor was scheduled for a herculean surgery to remove her primary tumor and the metastases in her right lung. The metastases were the "white spots" that the pulmonologist saw in her chest x-ray when we first found out Taylor had cancer. She had dozens of metastases, or tumors, in each lung, and the main tumor in the right lung had begun to invade and protrude into her airway. That was her "exercise-induced asthma." The tumors were restricting her lung capacity. Of course she had trouble on the soccer field. That's why this energetic young girl, who walked into Sloan, astonished the doctors.

During the pre-surgical conference, again only attended by Bob in an effort to shield and protect me, we both expected to hear the worst. Shockingly, Taylor's first oncologist, Dr. Redmond Sparrow, whose passive-aggressive personality was confusing and irritating, and our surgeon, Dr. Michael La Quaglia (also known as our hero), didn't agree on whether she should have surgery. The risks were enormous, and the surgery itself was life threatening. However, if the surgery wasn't performed, they told us, "Taylor's prognosis would likely be only a matter of months." What choice did we have? We thought the answer would be black and white and were stunned that the doctors presented Bob with their disagreements. Were they really asking Bob, a financier with no medical experience, to decide what to do with his daughter's life?

Their disagreements were both philosophy and medical. Many oncologists believe that if you haven't found a chemo or medicine that shrinks or kills the cancer, surgery that can't remove everything is unnecessary pain and risk for the patient. If you "can't get it all," it will merely continue to grow. Many believe it is better to keep trying medicines and/or focus on quality of life. Others don't.

Ultimately, the doctor's warnings about the risks of surgery fell on deaf ears. When we deciphered the medical jargon, it came down to this: If we did the surgery as planned, Taylor could possibly die on the table. If we didn't, we would lose her soon when the tumors took over. But if surgery were successful, we would buy time to keep trying. This was not, in the end, a hard decision, but it was agonizing.

We plowed forward at all costs with only one goal in mind: to save our daughter's life. A few days before surgery, a nurse called again to warn me of the risk. I rudely told her, "Never call again." I had heard enough!

I desperately wanted to know if Taylor understood the gravity of the surgery. I reached out to Amy, our favorite child life specialist at Sloan, a petite young woman whose never-ending energy and optimism always brightened our day. With fear rushing through my body, I asked, "Amy, I don't know if Tales thinks she could possibly not make it. I need your help!" Amy smiled, responding, "No problem, Sue."

Using props, Amy asked Taylor oodles of questions. To me, it seemed like they were playing with toys. I observed, said nothing, and felt totally clueless. Serious moments were intermingled with a lot of laughter. I later learned that Amy was using self-expression activities to interpret Taylor's feelings and was able to judge Taylor's reaction to her illness and upcoming surgery. Amy later explained to me, "Taylor has no thoughts of death, and she is feeling very supported." You can imagine the relief and gratitude I felt.

The day before surgery, Taylor mysteriously asked me to join her upstairs alone. A month or so prior, Taylor had asked, "Can you buy me sheet music to the song, 'My Heart Will Go On?'" known for its debut in the movie *Titanic*. I bought it for her, but after that I heard nothing about it. When I walked into the room, she sang to me, ever so tenderly, the words to the song that in essence asks the listener to carry on living after their loved one is gone.

I clenched the edge of my chair, my knuckles turning white. I feared Taylor could see my uncontrollable trembling as enormous tears slowly ran down my cheeks. Despite what Amy said, did Taylor think she might die? She was still a baby. Was she telling me it was okay, that no matter what our love would last a lifetime? Maybe she had overheard the repeated warnings and telephone calls from the nurses and doctors. I didn't know, and I was unwilling to ask her, so I willed myself to bury those thoughts. I smiled the best I could and listened to my angel tell me it was okay if she left us. Courage was second nature to her, but how she managed to sing that song to me is inconceivable. Whatever the outcome, she was going to make sure our love affair remained intact.

The Blackout

Taylor's surgery was looming just around the corner, like a dark shadow in the night, waiting to pounce and crush. Andrea had just arrived from North Carolina to pick up Ryan and Corey to stay with her during the surgery—thank God for her.

Ryan, Corey, and I hugged each other, refusing to separate, like little bear cubs with their mama. Tears cascaded down our faces, but neither of them complained. Ryan told me later, "I don't remember leaving or arriving in North Carolina. There are a lot of things that occurred during those years that I blocked out." It would have been easier if they had fought me about leaving; their silent, boundless courage made my heart ache. I waved goodbye and watched their car until I could see it no more. I dropped to my knees quivering, my body turning to ice.

I boarded the dogs at the kennel and cleaned our house from top to bottom. I can't imagine why I thought a clean house mattered, perhaps because it was something I could control when the rest of life seemed out of control. Two days later was Ryan's fourteenth birthday, the first birthday I would not spend with her. I knew in my heart that Andrea would make Ryan's birthday a big and memorable day, and she did, but I was crushed to miss it. Sometimes the whole series of events seemed to be one storm after another. This was no exception.

The night before surgery, Taylor, Bob, and I stayed at the Peninsula, located just west of Fifth Avenue in midtown Manhattan, a landmark Beaux-Arts building and a hotel we had been to several times before. Within minutes of being in the room, while Bob was parking the car, and as if my nerves weren't already frayed beyond capacity, the power suddenly went out. We were on a high floor and had no idea if there was a fire or if just our room had lost power, so we walked out into the hall—the elevators were not working. Taylor was terrified. In a panic, eyes wide, she exclaimed, "Can we go down the stairs right away, Mommy?"

As we rounded the corner of the dim stairwell, only to see more and more steps ahead, she cried, "Mommy, we could die!" Her words filled me with deep, raw emotions I didn't even know I had, and even worse, I had to keep them totally to myself because I didn't want to scare her. I knew we would make it down and be fine, but Taylor had no idea that her doctors had told us, "There is a very real possibility that Taylor might die on the operating table." My head spun as we made our way down the stairs that seemed to go on forever.

We arrived in the lobby to find out that all of New York City had gone black. The air was filled with angst, as we all wondered whether it was another terrorist attack. It was 2003 only two years post 9/11, when fears of terrorism were heightened in the United States, especially in New York City. As it turned out, it was the largest power outage in the history of North America (before Hurricane Sandy later claimed the title). Maybe it was just the timing, or maybe it was because I'm Italian and we're very superstitious, but I couldn't help but wonder if the blackout was an omen.

We called the hospital from a pay phone on the street, as there was no cell service. They reassured us, "Surgery is still a go. Don't worry, Mrs. Matthews; if the power isn't on in the morning, we have plenty of backup generators." Surgery was planned to be many hours. We thought, *Really? In a surgery where you may need to use any measure to keep Taylor alive, you want to use backup generators?* Nevertheless, we agreed, as this was back in the days when we still had complete blind faith in the medical world.

We had planned a beautiful evening with Taylor, including an extended visit to the wonderland of FAO Schwartz toy store on Fifth Avenue and a pizza dinner at her favorite Italian restaurant. That obviously wasn't happening now. Instead, Bob ran to the first deli he could find that was still open and grabbed handfuls of snacks. The snacks turned out to be a huge lifesaver. As many a chemo patient will attest, chemo destroys your taste buds and consequently causes your palate to change dramatically. Taylor had many assorted cravings, including snow cones, salami, and Oreos. If you couldn't find what she wanted when she wanted it, she became ugly. She told me, "Mommy, you don't understand what it's like to have chemotherapy. You really don't get it, and you're supposed to take care of me."

Thankfully, that night Bob had the wherewithal to act quickly and effectively, just like he always did. Many a time after Taylor was diagnosed, I would call Bob hysterical about the issue of the day, and he would listen calmly, put things in perspective, and respond with some form of, "I'm on the way."

As Tales tore open her snacks with the enthusiasm of a puppy dog with a bone, an ocean of tears welled deeply inside of me, threatening at any moment to spill over and betray my sorrow. I couldn't help but wonder, *Could this be Taylor's last dinner?* I wanted to vomit and rid myself of my pain, but to ease my pain I would've had to expel my very soul, which felt far darker than the blackened city that lay before me.

Somehow, we were able to get through to my sister and the girls in North Carolina. Scared, the girls cried, "Mommy and Daddy, we were so worried!" Andrea knew there was a chance Taylor might die in surgery the next day, because I had told her, but somehow she was able to keep them feeling safe with her.

Being out of town was the best thing for Ryan and Corey. Obviously, they were worried about their sister, but they were kids nonetheless. Bob and I always answered their questions honestly but did omit facts that were not age appropriate. They knew Taylor was having a massive surgery, but we didn't think that they needed to know, at ages nine and fourteen, that their sister could die. If we lost Taylor, knowing a day or so in advance wouldn't make it any easier for them. Not knowing allowed them to enjoy their time in a calm and soothing environment. And if we weren't willing to tell Taylor, how could we tell them?

The hotel management obliged Taylor by giving us a room on the first floor. As we waited for the key, my mind wandered to a time past when we stayed at the same hotel as a treat for the whole family. We went out for a nice dinner, and afterwards Taylor had her eye on a tray of chocolate truffles. Impatient with the waiter, she went over to the tray and, unbeknownst to us, filled her North Face jacket with the truffles and walked out of the restaurant, donning her signature smirk. The girls left the restaurant roaring with laughter as Taylor threw truffles in everyone's mouths, running down Fifth Avenue.

In complete darkness, we climbed a short flight of stairs up to our new room. The hotel was running on generators, with only emergency lights in the stairwells. The room felt eerie and ominous, in sharp contrast to the warm and inviting lobby whose glorious flowers never failed to impress. All we had was a small flashlight and the book *A Tree Grows in Brooklyn*, a favorite of my mother's. Taylor nestled into bed feeling safe and secure between both Bob's and my embrace, like this was just another adventure in her life. Throughout the evening, we took turns reading aloud. We couldn't see each other's faces, but I imagine deep worry lines permanently creased Bob's forehead that night, and extreme sadness weighed on him. Riddled with fear, we wanted nothing more than for time to stand still. Somehow, and only out of pure love for our daughter, we both maintained a sense of composure.

At approximately four in the morning, the power came back on. We got out of bed at five-thirty to arrive at our scheduled six o'clock appointment for surgery. All night I had had Taylor by my side through what felt like a wicked storm. Now the day had dawned, and we had to forge ahead, straight into the eye of the hurricane. I ran to the bathroom and vomited violently, my hands shaking so badly I could barely turn on the water faucet. How could I face the day, knowing by the end of it there was a chance my precious child would no longer be with us?

In the past, when we needed a distraction, Taylor and I used to drive around and sing the song "Leaving on a Jet Plane" by John Denver. Neither of us knew all the words, and I'm completely tone deaf, but we laughed and sang together. That song came to mind that morning. All I wanted to do was grab Taylor and make an escape, but indeed there was no dodging reality. Or so we thought.

We soon learned that only the west side of Manhattan had power. When we arrived at Sloan, on the east side, it was completely dark. We waited in the clinic, now dim and dirty from all the procedures performed the prior day. Food wrappers were strewn everywhere, sweaters that must've mistakenly been left behind hung on chairs, and a few blurry-eyed doctors roamed the floor, looking as if they had no purpose or destination. Eventually, they told us, "All surgeries are cancelled. We can reschedule Taylor in four days." As I began to sway, all I could wonder was, *Is God giving us four more days with Taylor before he takes her?* Dr. La Quaglia called from his car on the way in to the hospital and apologized for the delay, as if in some way he was responsible.

Little did we know, our ride home to Westchester would itself be death-defying. Just past 138th Street on the Bruckner Expressway, a major Manhattan highway with no shoulder, we got a flat rear tire. The dealership had a twenty-four-hour assistance number, but they were without power as well. There was no help coming, and we were trapped in the right lane with traffic flying past us.

Bob changed the tire as I frantically waved off cars. Rush hour approached, and we were in grave danger of being hit by the vehicles that continuously flew by, not realizing we were stopped. Taylor commented dryly, "I would much rather be under anesthesia than on this parkway." We laughed out loud. She always seemed to know how to relieve our tension.

We finally arrived home, and the house felt uncomfortably still. We headed out quickly to Lee's Art Store because Taylor said she wanted to buy supplies to make Christmas presents. It was August. Deep, dark thoughts invaded me. *Is Taylor making presents because she won't be with us in December?* The words "Taylor could die" echoed in my brain to the point where I felt trapped within myself. However, I still had my T for at least these few extra days, and I was determined not to squander them. At Taylor's request, we headed for Playland, the Westchester landmark amusement park, which all of our kids adored. Tales had a sense of the present at every turn. Given a moment to spend, she would make it fun.

As vivid as my memories are from the night before the original surgery date, I have no idea what we did the night before her rescheduled surgery date. I only remember Bob in his white "marshmallow" sterile suit the day of her surgery, complete with cap and covered shoes, ready to take Taylor into the operating room, or "OR." This would become our tradition: Bob would walk Taylor in and tell her, "I am the last person you will see when you close your eyes and the first person you see when you open them." Then he would stay with her until she fell asleep.

Tales didn't seem scared as she was prepped for surgery, but she was vigilant. She watched everyone like a hawk, answering every question precisely and insisting that people write down what she said. When the time came to head into the OR, Bob walked beside her and made idle conversation in an attempt to make her laugh. When he approached the OR doors, he asked, "Have you made up your mind about letting me help with the surgery?" He reminded them that he had worked in an emergency room at one point and deadpanned his fervent interest. Taylor shouted, "No, Daddy. Stop that!" She was giggling, but at the same time looking at the nurses and doctors to make sure they weren't taking him seriously.

She continued to watch Bob's eyes intently. I suppose she figured she didn't need to be scared if he wasn't. Of course, he never showed it, but Bob was terrified. He remembers that as they positioned her and put in the final IVs, she asked questions and giggled until they gave her Propofol, which knocked her out in seconds. "We laughed until she fell asleep," Bob told me later. "And then I begged the whole room to take special care of her, finally allowing my tears to flow freely."

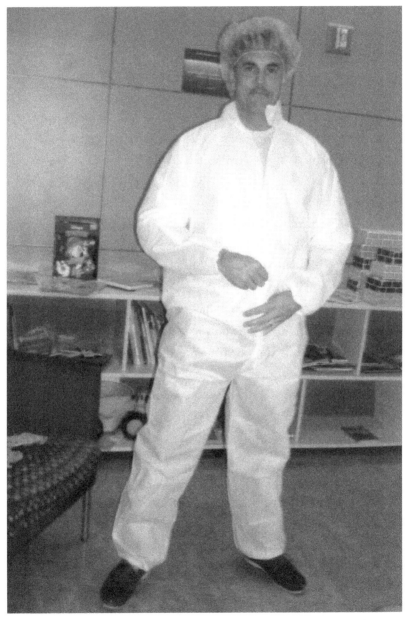

As for me, when they left for the OR, I completely fell apart, hysterically crying and barely able to breathe. Someone must have escorted me to the waiting area where, to my surprise, one of my dear friends and our school superintendent, Nancy, who made life for Taylor extraordinarily happy, was waiting for me. I had asked for no visitors, but Nancy said, "Sue, I just couldn't stay away." She calmly held me close. I felt like I was resting in the middle of a deep, soft cloud, and she just let me cry.

We waited and waited, every hour more excruciating than the one before. Coiled in my chair like a snake near a fire pit, I begged God to save Taylor. "But if you're going to take her," I implored, "please let her go in her sleep so she won't know." I wanted to spare my baby of her own death.

After *fourteen* hours, Dr. La Quaglia showed up in his street clothes, the picture of Cool Hand Luke—to tell us Taylor had made it!

In the recovery room, Taylor was hooked up to so many machines it was difficult to see her face, but when I did, she was barely recognizable. Her swelling was so severe it was hard to distinguish her nose from the rest of her face. Dr. La Quaglia reassured us by asking Taylor, "Can you wiggle your nose?" Wiggling her nose was a form of communication the two of them had set up as their private joke. She wiggled as best she could, and I breathed a deep breath for the first time all week.

Dr. La Quaglia is arguably the best pediatric oncology surgeon in the country. He is truly a legend.

Still, he has a gentle and calming manner and always engaged and reassured Taylor, even playing along with her pranks. Someone gave Taylor a bright yellow rubber chicken; Taylor wanted it in surgery with her, and he allowed it. The yellow chicken became a running joke between them. In his hands, we were assured that Taylor was never frightened and always believed all would be well. She feared no surgery that he was performing, an invaluable gift.

Amidst all the chaos, one of the doctors suddenly said, "We're moving Taylor to the ICU at Weill Cornell Medical Center across the street." At the time Sloan didn't have a pediatric ICU, but this was news to us. I screamed, "How can you do that? She needs a respirator to breathe!" Taylor also had two IV poles with four or five medicines running and several monitors measuring vital signs.

I momentarily checked out. It was as if a screen came down in front of me, separating me from the world, allowing me to distance myself as if I were watching a movie. Two supremely confident EMTs switched her to mobile versions of each monitor and pole and moved her to a stretcher for transport. They didn't flinch. Not a sign of fear. I remember being asked to sit in the front seat of the ambulance and hearing the driver tell me the cost of the ride to drive a quarter of a mile was $7,500. I stared blankly at him; his words were odd and garbled. Why was he telling me this?

Bob dashed across the street with our bags. When we arrived at Weill Cornell, they handled Taylor's stretcher indelicately to say the least. It was an extremely bumpy ride for a child still on life support. My motherly instincts kicked into overdrive. I wanted to shield my baby from this cruel and wicked world in which we now lived. Taylor whispered, "Mommy," to which I responded, "I'm here. I'm here, sweetheart." I have never in my life felt more like a mother than at that very moment. I was her lifeline.

The following day, I hit a wall, no longer able to keep my eyes open. Curled up in a chair and covered in blankets, I quickly fell into a deep, dreamless sleep. The anesthesiologists came to visit Taylor, and I was just waking up. Not noticing that I was under the ball of blankets on the chair, one doctor commented to another, "It's amazing what she tolerated. She lost almost the equivalent of her entire blood supply, and we were very lucky that the transfused blood flowed so rapidly to keep up with her blood loss." I suddenly arose, lurched forward, much to their surprise, and screamed, "What are you talking about? They didn't tell us that!" I learned in that moment the reality that many doctors intentionally omit information, only telling parents what they absolutely need to know. Nothing more.

During this surgery, Taylor's primary tumor, which had been located between her ribs, was removed. Afterwards, the doctors told us that during the operation they had decided, without consulting us, to refrain from placing a prosthesis where the tumor had laid, fearing it could cause infection. Consequently, an open space was left in her rib cage. We were furious that we were never given the opportunity to weigh in on the decision. The doctors simply didn't explain to us the possible side effects of leaving this open space, and as it turned out, leaving this hole was a problem just waiting to happen.

Taylor's recovery was nothing short of guts and fortitude. That was our Taylor—backbone made of steel, with a determination and grit to match. Tales was trying to "will" herself better. This proved extremely difficult for her and absolutely heartbreaking to watch. She was trying to tough it out, but it was not for the faint of heart. The pain management team struggled to manage her pain. I did a lot of praying, but truthfully, I was starting to wonder how God could allow an innocent child to suffer.

Then I remembered our three-day family trip to Shelter Island just one month ago. We had stayed at the Ram's Head Inn, a cozy bed and breakfast nestled among the forest-green trees right by the clear, blue water. Shortly after we arrived, I heard Taylor scream, "Mommy, I keep on asking God to make it better, and it only gets worse!" Her words pierced me like the end of a sharp knife. How I fetched my response, I will never know. I quoted words from the poem "Footprints in the Sand," by Margaret Fishback Powers which teaches you that when you only see one set of footprints that is because God is carrying you.

Taylor hung on to those words in her heart and later said, "Throughout my treatments, it has helped knowing that God is always protecting me and carrying me while I am sick."

My niece Samantha tells me, "God doesn't *cause* suffering, but He does *allow* it. It's all part of His master plan." I go back and forth on that one. It's easy to say things like "have faith" and "everything happens for a reason" until you witness your own flesh and blood writhe in a kind of excruciating pain you never knew or imagined existed.

Mischief on 68th Street

After several very scary days immediately following her surgery, Taylor seemed to be perking up, especially for a kid who had been hacked apart days earlier. She was moved back across from the ICU at Weill Cornell to the Step Down at Sloan. Tubes, wires, and IVs hung everywhere. Every mandatory walk down the hall was a major logistical effort of switching to mobile units and arranging medical and physical support, while enduring a whole lot of pain.

Anyone working in a surgical unit knows that preventing complications from surgery and jumpstarting one's recovery requires getting the patient out of bed and mobile as soon as possible. From the very first moment Taylor could stand the pain and bear the risk, she was walking. She didn't like it, and she didn't do it without protest. Getting her to walk against her wishes took more than pronouncement; it took intense negotiation and persuasion. Telling Taylor what to do was the surest way to ensure it would not happen. Donald Trump would have been easier to negotiate with. And so it came to be that Taylor, after significant detente, agreed to three walks around the floor for the day.

It was still August; the weather was warm, and the city was quiet. Sun washed the floor in her hospital room at the end of the day. Taylor was exhausted and irritable about being cooped up. Every twenty minutes or so, the nurses would pop in, saying, "Remember, Taylor; you owe us one more walk." Taylor would listen, wave them off, and turn her head.

On the last attempt, the senior nurse came to push Taylor—and push her hard. She played the integrity card: "Taylor, you promised one more walk today." The nurse tried to make the walk sound appealing by suggesting that Taylor walk outside for some fresh air. Taylor was uncharacteristically immune to the nurse's appeal. She was done with demands and pushing. She turned away again. The nurse looked to Bob for an assist. He told the nurse, "Leave it to me." He knew his audience.

Bob very gently put his hand on Taylor's head, and as she turned toward him, he said, "Tales, you know this is part of getting back on your feet and getting home. You promised one more walk. I know you have had it with the pain and the pushy people. But I think you're missing an opportunity." Her eyes searched his for a hint.

"Tales," he said, "they want a walk? Let's give them a walk they'll never forget." She was intrigued. He had her attention now and could see her impish grin. "They think we should go outside? Let's go outside!" Taylor began giggling, knowing she was part of a scheme created by Bob. "Tales," he said, "let's go get some ice cream!" Tales was as energized and as upbeat as she had been in a while.

Since I wasn't there at the time, Bob told me all about it later. "She fidgeted, while suppressing her giggles and excitement as they mundanely moved the IV lines, disconnected the wires, and set up the mobile IV pole." The nurses couldn't believe her change in enthusiasm. They waved and called out, "You go, girl! Take your time and walk as much as you like!" Tales didn't hear a word. She was laboring, tired, and in pain, but she was giddy. She was on a mission.

When the elevator opened on the ground floor, Tales headed for the main entrance onto York Avenue. Bob remembers the smell of cigarette smoke filling his nose as they passed a pack of hospital patients getting some air—most of them, unbelievably, smoking. Taylor never noticed or flinched. She skillfully kept walking, turning left at the corner of 68th Street and heading uphill toward First Avenue. This was one heck of a walk!

Tales was still in her hospital gown, a thin gray smock with the back wide open, exposing blood seeping through the bandages. Her underwear was like a flag waving in the back as she pushed her IV pole laden with three bags. She looked to any passersby like an escapee from a mental institution, and Bob remembers thinking that they wouldn't have been completely wrong. But this was New York City, home of the good, the bad, and the ugly, and a half-naked insane person strutting down the street wasn't that shocking.

She should have been afraid of the uphill walk and the physical effort, but instead she was delighted at calling the shots and once more poking her finger in the eye of the giant. People on the street stopped, stared, and then applauded. Cabs tooted their horns, maybe thinking she was a nut or maybe congratulating her. Passengers opened windows to cheer her. They all laughed like it was a publicity stunt. She walked all the way up that hill, huffing and puffing, turned right onto First Avenue, and kept walking. First Avenue is far busier than York Avenue, so there was even more commotion. Taylor was clearly tired but elated and felt in control.

The truth is, neither Bob nor Taylor knew exactly where the ice cream store was, and there was no such thing as Siri in 2003. Bob asked Taylor, "Do we turn left or right?" They weren't sure how far they had to go, but really, this wasn't about the ice cream. They were taking a walk, Taylor style.

Bob watched as sweat accumulated on Taylor's brow and she began to look a little pale. Her little body was asking for a break. He could see that her steps were slowing, and she was leaning on the pole, which he was now pushing. The point was made. The ice cream seemed to get farther away with each step. She was still smiling and enjoying the street attention, but she was ready to go back to her bed for some care and monitoring. Bob said, "This was the plan all along—take the walk, make a point, and return triumphantly, demonstrating who was in control." Adventure over. Taylor, 1; hospital, 0.

Downhill was obviously easier, and I'm sure she felt more secure knowing she was on the way back toward comfort and care. What Bob didn't know was that the nursing staff had begun to panic. After all, a post-surgical patient can only walk so far. The nurses started asking the patients on the street, "Did you see a young girl passing by?" I guess someone recalled her "turning left a while ago." Now they really hit the panic button. Security was called, and a search was initiated. They were missing a very sick patient who was under their care.

Around that time, I received a call on my cell phone and heard a very angry voice ask me, "Do you know where your daughter is? She has been off the floor for a significant amount of time, and, Mrs. Matthews, you do understand how sick she is!" I asked, "Who are you?" The person on the other end declared, in an arrogant and aggressive tone, "This is security!" I replied, calmly and perhaps a little smugly, "Yes, I understand she is very ill, but if she is with her dad, I am sure all is well." Of course, this only infuriated them more.

In the meantime, Bob and Tales were gliding downhill toward York Avenue when suddenly they saw two very angry security guards trudging up the hill. Laughing, Bob said, "These guys weren't exactly physical specimens, so the hill was no bargain for them. They were sweating more than Tales was. And they were clearly out of breath."

Watching two very perturbed and portly security guards running uphill looking for her was the perfect end to the walk. The more she laughed, the angrier the guards got, until they finally reached her. By now, anyone could look at the scene and put some of this together. Those watching whooped or gave her a thumbs-up. The guards chuckled, too. It was hard not to laugh along with Bob and Taylor. Bob remembers Tales being in her glory as she strolled past the security guards with her head held high.

Two very pissed-off nurses were waiting when they got back to her hospital floor. Tales tried not to antagonize them and painstakingly held in her laughter, but both she and Bob looked like the proverbial "cats who ate the canary," sporting huge grins. Neither of them spoke a word as Bob tried not to look at the nurses. He knew at whom they were really mad. The head nurse blurted out, "Where have you been?" and that was all Tales could take. The giggles took over, and all she could get out was "ice cream." She kept walking. Bob kept walking. The nurses trailed behind, clearly feeling dismissed. As they glared at Bob, looking for an explanation, he just held his hands up with a shrug, saying, "She took a walk, just like you asked." Uncharacteristically, Tales said nothing. She was triumphant but clearly running on fumes.

Moving her to the bed and re-establishing all of her wires and tubes was done with a constant drone of criticism for taking such risks and worrying everyone. Sometimes it was directed at Bob and sometimes at Taylor. Tales just smiled, but the nurses were starting to hit a nerve. She glanced at them with her "you're boring me" look and said, "I'm sorry you were so worried, but my dad was with me. You told me I could walk as much as I wanted, and you told me I could go outside. So, I did." She turned away and closed her eyes, as she reached for Bob's hand.

Instantly Bob felt warm all over, as emotion and pride rose up and pulsated throughout his veins. As she held his hand, he knew how much she appreciated him taking her on their adventure and that she was glad he was staying with her that night. But he couldn't help but think that by not letting his hand go, she was also protecting him from the nurses who were anxious to have a private word with him. She was fast asleep in minutes, clearly wiped out and exhausted. But she never let go.

Bob tells me that sometimes when he closes his eyes, he can still feel her hand in his.

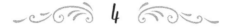

4

A New Normal

We cannot change the cards we are dealt,
just how we play the hand.

–Randy Pausch

Laughter Is the Best Medicine

After a fourteen-hour operation and a week of chemotherapy that kept Tales hospitalized for five weeks, she was exhausted, in pain, nauseous, and missing home. She had lost all her senses, living in a world of recirculated air. I knew, even at her worst, instead of just sleeping, she needed a diversion to make her happy and feel challenged. At times, I felt like a kindergarten teacher, always looking for the next activity to keep her busy.

I thought of Amy, our wonderful child life specialist, and Mary, Taylor's favorite nurse, and enlisted their help. Mary was not only Taylor's nurse but also her dear friend and companion. Whenever she was sad, she would find Mary who would instantly brighten her day.

Amy knew that Taylor was an artist. Taylor had taken up oil painting when she gave up sports due to her illness. She absolutely loved it, once commenting, "In some ways, having cancer is a blessing because I would've never become an artist." *Really, Tales?* I thought. It was hard to believe she actually spoke those words. Amy asked, "Taylor, would you like to paint something for display for Pediatric Cancer Awareness Month?" Taylor was thrilled with the concept and quickly agreed to help out.

As much as she wanted to paint, it was heartbreakingly difficult for her to do so. Her ability to write or raise her arm was still temporarily impaired due to surgery. Instead, she issued orders and I executed them, which was, come to think of it, nothing unusual. Amy hung a large white canvas on the wall in her room. Taylor envisioned a large gold ribbon, symbolizing pediatric cancer, with multi-colored handprints all around it. Taylor named the piece "Hold the Hand of a Child," clearly expressing her need to be held. I wrote the words and painted the gold ribbon while she supervised.

"Mommy, can we use both of our handprints on the canvas?"

"Of course," I replied as I lifted her out of bed and put her in a wheelchair. She was too weak to walk across the hospital room, which was maybe four steps. She dipped her hands inside the paint buckets with the same smile she had in nursery school when fun was about to begin. I ever so gently held her arms and hands up so she could reach the canvas. She loved it, beaming the entire time. She always found fun at every corner. A day of pure fun while in the midst of chemotherapy was a godsend.

Taylor's protocol called for a series of different chemotherapies repeated on a precise schedule. She was due to receive a particularly harsh chemotherapy that she had had for the first time two months prior. The first time she had this chemo, she had mouth sores that extended from her mouth all the way down her esophagus. Sobbing to me, she said, "Mommy, drinking water feels like I'm drinking glass." It hurt so much to watch; I can only imagine what it felt like to Tales.

Again, we couldn't control her chemo, but we could control having fun. Now, I had to dig deep into my Mom bag of tricks to distract her. She was angry at the disease, the doctors, the nurses, and Bob and me. And we felt guilty for what we were doing to her. Suddenly, it hit me: Taylor needed to let her anger out. I grabbed two-dozen eggs, ran to our backyard, and Tales fired away. Bob and I threw them back at her, but her aim was far more effective, and she didn't mind putting some zip on her throws. She laughed in the same infectious way we loved. All of us were dripping with egg goo in our hair and on our clothes while laughing our butts off. As Erma Bombeck says, "Laughter rises out of tragedy; when you need it most, it rewards you with courage." Taylor's tension melted from her body like ice on a hot day. She couldn't fathom that I had actually suggested this activity. Let's just say I've been called a "neat freak" in my day.

Although I thought we had cleaned everything up, the following day both of our dogs were sick from eating raw eggs. They were vomiting egg goo while Taylor was vomiting from chemotherapy. Though miserable, Taylor thought it was hilarious that I spent the day cleaning up vomit. A little bit of craziness can really go a long way.

Another time, when Taylor had had it, I called Amy again, and in what seemed like an instant, she appeared carrying buckets of paint and balloons. Just the sight of her cracked us up; it hardly mattered what she had planned! Amy handed us funny, thin yellow paper gowns, often seen around the hospital, and balloons filled with paint, and she taped a plastic sheet onto the wall. Next thing you know, we were throwing the paint-filled balloons as hard as we could until they burst on the walls. Splat! Taylor's anxiety gave way to laughter, and the smile on her face melted me on the spot.

An Unusual Sleepover

When someone in the family gets cancer, the whole family gets cancer. On many evenings, Corey and Ryan were home alone while I was inpatient with Taylor. Beata would leave for the day at seven o'clock, and because my two beauties insisted they didn't want someone to live with us, they were alone until Bob could get home. Abandoning them would've been a lot less painful if today's technology had existed. Things we now take for granted, like FaceTime, allow families to be more united. In those days without smartphones, when we were sequestered in the hospital, I could call but never physically see the girls, nor could they see Taylor. If seeing Taylor was a possibility, a lot of fear could have been alleviated. Taylor also likely would have been much happier if she had had access to social media.

One night, missing me terribly, my little Corey decided to spend the night with us in the hospital. Even though it was strictly prohibited, we needed each other. The room had two patients in it, separated by a thin multi-colored curtain. Our side of the room had a leather pullout couch that slept two, a hospital bed, and all the hospital accompaniments, including IV poles, blood-pressure monitors, and boxes of sterile rubber gloves. Not the best place for a sleepover, but we didn't care.

Every night, Taylor slept with me on the pullout couch, leaving her bed vacant. This night was no different: Tales was not about to give up her spot alongside her mommy to Corey. She was so sick that I agreed—although now I feel some regret, because it was the one night Corey could've snuggled with me. Late that night, Corey fell into a deep slumber in Taylor's hospital bed. Taylor had slept all day, so even though it was the middle of the night, we got up and went into a nearby lounge. Day and night were becoming indistinguishable. When the nurses came to check vitals, they failed to notice Corey's thick, long hair sprawled on the pillowcase and thought she was Taylor. When they woke Corey up, she screamed and darted out into the hallway, not knowing where we were or what to do. When she found Taylor and me in the lounge, she was enraged. "Mommy!" she cried. "They thought I was a cancer patient, and they woke me up! I was so scared, Mommy! Where were you? Why weren't you there?" It may not have been what Corey had envisioned when she signed on for a sleepover, but it was better than spending yet another night apart.

We're Not in Kansas Anymore

Taylor was scheduled for a second thoracotomy, three days before Halloween and four days before her twelfth birthday. We moved up her birthday party but tried to be realistic: "Tales, there is a very good chance you will be in the hospital on Halloween and your birthday." She took one look at us and emphatically replied, with requisite attitude and sass, "I'll make it out!" Our bets were always on Taylor, but this time we had considerable doubt and were no longer taking disappointments very well.

All systems were in place for a last-minute birthday bash. The concept of over-the-top kids' birthday parties rose to new heights. However, if we were going to go a little overboard, this year was the time to do it. Aunt Andrea came up for a week-long visit in advance of Taylor's party, making everything one long celebration.

We planned a murder mystery birthday party, a la Agatha Christie, hosting seventy kids at Sleepy Hollow Country Club, whose main house is a former Vanderbilt family estate built in the late 1800s, a perfect venue for the intrigue that would follow. Twenty kids and Andrea's best friend Danielle, who had a background in theater, were selected in advance and given parts as "suspects," with roles to play, costumes, and clues.

I called on a dear friend, Barbara, whose adoring blue eyes and kind heart always made Taylor smile. Barbara was ever-present in Taylor's life and helped us tremendously at every curve, and this time was no different. She worked tirelessly prior to the party, making sure the kids got their roles and fielding the many questions they had. Taylor was "Jessica Fletcher" and led the investigation. Everyone had to figure out "whodunit," and the kids all loved it. Taylor even wore a wig under a knit hat for the first and only time.

Shortly after the birthday party, Taylor had her second thoracotomy. Thankfully, it was a success. A couple dozen more tumors were removed from our child's lungs. Unfortunately, Dr. La Quaglia told us, many remained; he couldn't get them all.

We were infinitely grateful to Dr. La Quaglia and felt relieved when it was over, but afterwards the nurses forbade us from going to the recovery room to see Taylor. Instead, they forced us to wait in her hospital room, which had never happened before. After major surgery, can you imagine your child waking up to a stranger? We were appalled and decided we would no longer play by the rules. This would never happen again! Our fears were confirmed when Taylor was finally wheeled into her room, quaking with terror, a look of panic screaming through her crying eyes. To make matters worse, they did not give her any anti-nausea medication, despite our insistence that, based upon her history after the last surgery, she would need it.

The next day started off on a good note when the doctors agreed to take out her chest tube. Imagine a rubber hose the diameter of your pinky inserted into a hole cut into your side near the ribs. It hurt coming out, but not as much as it hurt staying in. Surprisingly, Taylor also insisted on weaning off her IV pain medication, even though she needed it. We soon realized this was part of her plan all along, but none of us understood her strategy until Taylor's now primary oncologist, Dr. Bill Oscar, visited.

He entered her room, hands clasped behind his back, sporting his typical frown. His mood was hard to judge, as his creased forehead and grumpy scowl seemed permanently etched on his face. The decision about when Taylor could go home was up to Dr. La Quaglia, but we knew Dr. Oscar, the ultimate curmudgeon, was never on her side and would be adding his two cents. His arrogance was astounding. Every time he walked in the room, we didn't know whether an earthquake was coming or a volcano was about to erupt, but the air around us definitely shifted.

Without expression, he asked Taylor, "How are you feeling?" to which she sweetly but confidently replied, "Pretty well. I'm leaving on Friday, on Halloween." Not surprisingly, he threw his arms in the air and grunted, "That's impossible: you still have a chest tube; you need oxygen and IV pain medication." Taylor proudly asked him to come to the side of her bed. She watched his expression, with great satisfaction, as he noticed that she no longer had a chest tube or an IV pain pump. Instead of congratulating her, he glared at her and responded, "You still need oxygen," and condescendingly left the room.

As if we didn't know already, this was complete affirmation that someone with an ego as large as his, and virtually zero bedside manner, would not be Taylor's doctor for long. We also understood what was coming next. Taylor had made a decision. Step in her path at your own risk.

Ryan and Corey arrived at the hospital that evening with bags of Halloween decorations. Corey reassured Taylor in a soothing voice, "Don't worry, Tales; we're going to make Halloween just as awesome here as it always is at home." They turned Taylor's room into a Halloween scene that resembled a set from Broadway. Their talents were immeasurable, but the warmth, love, and compassion they showed their sister that evening took my breath away. Taylor beamed with joy.

I had no idea what Halloween looked like at home this year or what my little Corey was wearing for a costume. I knew we had the best babysitter, Beata, whose big green eyes reflected her inner warmth, and that she would take care of everything, but like any nine-year-old, Corey wanted her mommy. My emotions burned my throat like scorching acid. But I had to swallow it. None of this was lost on Taylor. She apologized many a time for taking me away from Ryan and Corey.

Before cancer, excitement abounded when my three little ones watched the Halloween boxes come up from the basement. Within seconds, the couch was filled with Halloween-themed stuffed animals and decor. The witches were placed in the kitchen (I guess this was a hint, because they hated my cooking). The girls would run to the phone, asking, "Daddy, when are we carving our real pumpkins?" Of course, we also had singing pumpkins, goblins, and, the family favorite, a singing witch hat. In past years, Halloween could not only be seen but also heard throughout our home—and maybe even down the street.

Coming up with an idea for a costume for Taylor while living in the hospital was no easy undertaking, especially because there were no smartphones or Wi-Fi enabled laptops in those days. Taylor went to the hospital playroom to use their desktop computers, which meant some rest time for me, time to regroup and get ready for whatever was to come next. We were living moment to moment.

Suddenly, Taylor barreled into the room: "Mommy, I figured out a costume!" She had printed a huge picture of the candy label "Jelly Belly." She snatched a large, clear hospital garbage bag and asked urgently, "Can you run to the hospital gift shop to get balloons in every color?" She glued the label on the garbage bag, put her legs through the bottom, filled the garbage bags with the balloons, and tied the opening around her neck. She squealed, "Ryan, can you find red tights and bring in my red hat?" She bounced around the hospital hallways dressed as a bag of jellybeans! The only thing brighter than her costume was the smile on her face. If fun didn't find Taylor, Taylor would find the fun.

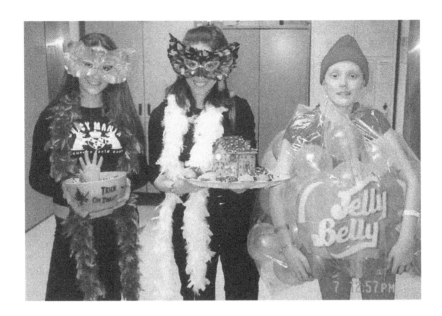

As the two of us were sitting outside Taylor's room on low stools, making spider webs out of white gooey string, Dr. La Quaglia came for a visit and asked very gently, "Tales, how are you feeling?" She robustly replied, "Okay, ready to leave!" Halloween was the next day. He bowed his head and looked at both of us with great sadness in his eyes. "Tales, you still need oxygen, so you can't go home." Taylor quickly turned her face away. He was officially being shunned.

I could see the tears suddenly cascading down her face; she was embarrassed to let Dr. La Quaglia see her cry. When I attempted to comfort her, she pushed me away. She could endure physical pain but not this. She had tried everything she could to escape in the past few days and suffered greatly for it. Her body shrunk, and her eyes became dark and distant. Suddenly, it seemed there was no fight left in her, a very different picture from the daughter I saw fighting all week to get better.

Taylor knew Dr. La Quaglia was hurting as badly as she was. He had a compassion and warmth for Taylor that was remarkable, but he was letting her down. Bob often said, "Letting Tales down was unbearable for anyone who participated with her in her battle." The hallway was filled with gut-wrenching silence as the three of us sat there, surrounded by Halloween spider webs. It was as if the webs had trapped Taylor in a cocoon, and there was no escape.

I tried to think rationally while feeling totally irrational. I asked Dr. La Quaglia, "Is oxygen the only thing keeping her here?" He nodded his head yes in defeat. Not knowing much about our options, I begged, "Can we get portable tanks at home? I can monitor her." I could hear the despair in his voice as he whispered, "It will take social services a day or two to get authorization."

That was an answer I could work with. "If I can get the tanks tomorrow, will you allow her to go home?" He nodded his head yes while eyeing Tales. Atypically, Tales never looked at him again as he stood up, ready to go. We exchanged glances. I nodded with a small smile as he turned to walk away. Taylor's silence was very troubling. I immediately told her, "I will get the oxygen, and you will go home." Again, she pushed me aside, pulled her oxygen tank, and got into bed. I followed her and tried to hug her, with no response.

The social workers had left for the evening. I found the head nurse and explained my predicament. She showed compassion but stated, "There is nothing I can do at night. We'll look into it tomorrow morning, but it's virtually impossible to get oxygen in one day." My sadness turned to rage. I exploded, "We are talking about oxygen, not a medical procedure! This is purely about logistics, and after all my daughter has suffered, *you will* find a way to make this work!"

She scowled and, without a word, walked away. Really? I ran to follow her and screamed, "We are on a pediatric oncology ward, and you are heartless!" I knew screaming was not going to help, and maybe she was just doing her job, but I couldn't help myself. I was infuriated and, quite frankly, so out of my mind that I have no memory of anything else that happened afterwards that evening. I don't remember if I even slept that night, but I got a call from Beata early the next morning: "The oxygen tanks are here."

Taylor left the hospital, but she was still in pain, still laboring for breath, still too weak to walk house to house with her friends. Meanwhile, as all of this was unfolding, Bob was searching for a blockbuster birthday present. He'd come up with an idea, but it was a bit far-fetched and more than a small challenge logistically. He bought Taylor a Segway, a little electric stand-up scooter that moves by shifting your body weight. It can transport you up to three times a normal walking pace and start, stop, and turn on a dime. They were 2003's version of today's hoverboards, only they had handles.

The problem was, the only dealer we could find was in Southampton, New York, on the tip of Long Island. That did not stop Bob. His good friend Jim, who would do anything for Tales and who was probably her first crush, drove all the way out to the Hamptons to get it. When she arrived home and saw it, Taylor seemed to bounce from the floor right up to the ceiling, eyes like giant saucers, exclaiming, "This is the best present *ever*! When can we try it?" It was now dark outside, so she rode it around the house giggling as she banged into walls and furniture. The gift wasn't just about a cool toy. It ensured that Tales had mobility.

She would, indeed, celebrate Halloween, and she would, indeed, go trick-or-treating in her jellybean costume with a twenty-foot-long oxygen tube in her nose tucked in a bag on the Segway. Afterwards, she did some candy swapping and hung out at her friend Allie's, like any normal twelve-year-old kid would. Cancer, be damned!

Around the same time, I received a call from my girlfriend Jeanne, a friend of twenty-five years. Jeanne, with her thick blonde hair and tiny frame, looks delicate, but she is fierce and the ultimate caregiver, the ever-ready battery who never stops trying to care for others.

"Sue, what? Taylor has cancer? Why didn't you tell us? We're devastated. What can we do?"

By "we" she meant herself, Lori, and Barbara, all dear friends from my working days at Deloitte. We had lost touch, given all that had happened following diagnosis. I was functioning at one-hundred miles an hour, putting out fires and never sleeping for more than three consecutive hours, but it hit hard to realize I had neglected to call dear friends months after diagnosis. It frightened me to think there could be other important things I was forgetting.

The next day was Taylor's birthday. As I watched her open her gifts, I let my mind wander to a year ago, her last birthday pre-cancer, but found I didn't remember much. Even then, just a few months after diagnosis, I feared my memories were fading. My mind was mush.

I looked at a photograph taken on Taylor's last birthday. Sliding my fingers across the picture, I desperately wanted to feel, breathe, touch, and relive that moment, just for a second. I could see Taylor's eyes twinkling. I was wearing a big, fluffy, bright-green robe, whose familiar comfort I hadn't felt in a long time. I saw the joy in my eyes, and all of a sudden, reality assaulted me. I desperately wanted my life back. With tears streaming, I wondered, *Did Taylor have cancer then?* No one will ever know.

Tales was honored with another thrilling surprise for her birthday. Our neighbors arranged for the charitable organization Songs of Love to write a song about Taylor and record it professionally. Everybody and everything that was important in Taylor's life made it into the song: her family, her best friends, and her favorite belongings. The music and lyrics are all original. We couldn't stop listening to it or singing the chorus, "Everything's okay if I'm with Tay!"

Later that day, my sister Lynn had something extra special planned. She orchestrated her own production of *The Wizard of Oz*, complete with costumes, scripts, and music, right in our vestibule. My father was the Cowardly Lion, Taylor was Dorothy, Uncle Bill was the Tin Man, and Lynn, ironically, was Glinda, the good witch. It was a great day, although Lynn complained afterwards that I didn't "thank her" enough for her efforts. My life was a complete whirlwind, so maybe I didn't. Who knows? All I can say is, the whole thing couldn't have been more appropriate, because we certainly weren't in Kansas anymore.

Accidental Overdose

Following her very aggressive second lung surgery, Taylor was in considerable pain. Painkillers were a part of her everyday life. I kept a journal listing every dose of medication that she was given and painstakingly reviewed each dose before I administered it.

At the same time, I was exhausted and still fighting every day to make sense of the fact that Taylor had cancer. One day, harried and distracted, I gave the job of handing out the pain medication to Bob. He recited the instructions: "One of these and two of those." But he was also wiped out and got the dosages backward. "Wait, Bob; you gave her what?" I screamed. Bob was truly scared. He had made a dreadful mistake, resulting in an accidental overdose of Oxycodone.

It was evening and Taylor was feeling fine, not acting any differently and having a grand time telling stories with Aunt Andrea, Ryan, and Corey. After watching and speaking with her, we thought, "Okay, no big deal," and I almost didn't call the hospital. What world was I living in? The pre-cancer world, where things were normal and there wasn't a fire drill every other week. Andrea told me later, "So many times when I was visiting, I'd say goodnight and go to sleep, assuming all was well—only to awaken the next morning and learn of three different emergencies that had come up overnight. I honestly have no idea how you functioned without sleep." The branches of cancer life kept strangling and entangling us to the point where there was virtually no rest at all.

In the end, I called the doctor. He admonished me and said, "Come in *immediately*." It was around ten at night, and we lived forty-five minutes away from the hospital. We had all just put on our pajamas and were settling in, exhausted. I argued, "But, Taylor looks and feels fine," to which the doctor replied, "Mrs. Matthews, you don't understand the gravity of the situation." I wanted to live life on my terms, but his words and his tone sent me packing our overnight bag without further hesitation.

As I approached Taylor's room to tell her the news, I could hear bursts of laughter, as animated stories were being exchanged between Aunt Andrea and my girls. Still a child herself, Taylor didn't think about yesterday or worry about tomorrow. She lived in the moment, and in that moment, she was immensely happy. For Taylor, this was usually a saving grace, but on this night, it worked against her.

I dreaded telling Taylor she had to be admitted to the hospital. Bob was guilt ridden. With distant, heartsick eyes, I finally confessed, "We overdosed you on your meds. We have to go to the hospital now." She clung to her aunt while bracing herself against the sides of her sandy-brown wooden sleigh bed. With tears of disbelief streaming down her face, she screamed at me, "This is *not* fair; Aunt Annie is leaving tomorrow! I'm *not* going to the hospital, Mommy!" The two of them held each other tightly, crying like little girls. Ryan and Corey's eyes showed their deep sadness, but they had become used to Taylor having to go back to the hospital on the flip of a dime.

Taylor was admitted to the Step-Down Unit of the ICU, where she was monitored intently. In the morning, after Taylor had a great night's sleep, I asked, "Why are syringes tied to Taylor's IV pole?" The nurse barked, with angry eyes, "Mrs. Matthews—or should I say, *Doctor* Matthews—you significantly overdosed your daughter. She may have needed resuscitation." I was shocked. The seriousness of the situation hadn't hit me, I suppose, because it all worked out fine. For me, the real tragedy of the situation still was pulling Taylor away from home that night, a home she was holding on to for dear life.

Driving Outside the Lines

We had been in cancer hell for only a few months, but it already felt like an eternity. "This is a jail sentence, Mommy! How can they make me stay home?" whined Taylor. Thanks to chemotherapy, Taylor had a low immune system, a condition called neutropenia, which made it incredibly difficult to fight off infections. Staying away from all germs meant public places were forbidden and visitors were limited. Try explaining that to a twelve-year-old with ants in her pants.

With slumped shoulders, she looked defeated as she sluggishly walked over to her favorite blue and yellow striped chair in our family room. "Well, why don't you just eat a sleeve of Oreos?" I offered. Her face brightened. She knew Oreos weren't healthy, and for her entire life, I was one of those moms who harped on eating well. However, according to the "cancer rules," when one doesn't have an immune system, the more processed the food, the safer it is. Intuitively, that makes no sense to me, but I went with it.

The Oreo feast calmed Taylor but for only a few minutes. I thought, "Damn it, Sue; why don't you have a plan for the day?" Again, I was the kindergarten teacher, but my options were limited.

Demoralized, Taylor slumped into her chair, grabbed the remote, and put on *ER* reruns. It beggared my heart to see Taylor watch television, something she rarely did before she got sick. Chemotherapy had taken over; her energy was low, and she appeared to be giving in to her situation.

I grabbed her books from the car, thinking that getting some schoolwork done would be distracting and productive. Taylor gave me one of her "are you serious, and now I might stab you" looks. Suddenly, it came to me. I turned around, threw her books right back into the car, and ran into the house with excitement. "Taylor, do you want me to teach you how to drive?" I smiled and laughed, waiting for her to process what I had just said. She looked up, confused at first, and then her face could have illuminated the entire block.

Taylor screamed with pure delight, "Let's go!" She threw a coat over her pajamas and sprinted to the car as if she were an exceptionally trained racehorse. My veins were pulsing, my heart throbbing. I was breaking into a cold sweat as both anxiety and excitement crept up my spine. I knew Taylor would be fearless, gutsy, and cocky behind the wheel. Yet my trepidation was overshadowed by my elation at being able to give Taylor a gift, a gift I had control over at a time when we had no control.

Taylor's expression of pure jubilance filled me with a surreal feeling. She was back again, wild as ever, ready for the next adventure. My car was parked in the middle bay of our garage, with steel poles surrounding each side.

"Tales, I think Mommy should pull the car out of the garage."

"No way," she answered, reminding me of the time I sideswiped our brand-new gray Murano the first time I pulled into the garage. "You did that after driving for twenty-five years. I'm staying in the driver's seat."

Taylor carefully and very slowly backed the car out. I sighed, thinking, *At least she is being cautious.* That lasted all of two seconds. She blasted down the driveway and through our cul-de-sac on the correct side of our tree-lined center island. Taylor got to the end of our street, ready to make a right turn onto Underhill Road, a fairly busy thoroughfare. I screamed, "Are you crazy? You are only driving on *our* street." She agreed and made a U-turn, heading back in the direction of our home. I sighed with relief.

But instead of pulling into our driveway, she turned around again, drove down the street, and, with her tiny nose peering over the driver's seat, had the nerve this time to actually turn onto Underhill Road before I could stop her. I grabbed the sides of my seat, looked both ways, took a deep breath, and went completely silent, desperately wanting to close my eyes but unable to blink. It was not as easy as she expected, but we did get home safely. As we roared up the driveway, she said, with her signature devilish smile, "I'm pulling the car into the garage, *Susssan,*" and she did, without missing a beat.

Thereafter, it was game on; Taylor drove all the time. I know it was crazy and irresponsible. But there was something about the rebellion that invigorated us.

Who was going to stop me, a mother with a bald child next to her in the car? I actually daydreamed of *daring* someone to do so.

I realized, after the fact, that Ryan, being the oldest, might legitimately object to Taylor's learning how to drive first, but I was so desperate I couldn't reverse course. Ryan, consistent with her patient, understanding character, never made a fuss. Knowing my uneasiness, Ryan would say, "It's fine, Mommy. I understand." But I think it bothered her greatly. In retrospect, I should have known that inequities amongst my girls hurt, no matter the circumstances.

One of our hardest hurdles continued to be making sure our other girls didn't get overlooked, both literally and emotionally. Ryan and Corey consistently got shortchanged, while also feeling guilty as the "lucky" healthy children. But there was nothing lucky about having a sick sister, losing your full-time stay-at-home mom to the hospital, and having to listen to your dad softly crying at night as he clicked away on the computer keyboard, searching for answers.

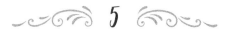

5

One Hundred Blocks Uptown

Medicine is aptly described as an art, not a science.

–Andrew Saul

I'll Be Home for Christmas

Life has a way of keeping your priorities in order. When pediatric cancer patients surround you, you realize pretty quickly that there's no time like the present. Taylor launched into the Christmas season like a gale-force wind. She was determined to observe every tradition and take every opportunity to celebrate. Not a minute was squandered.

Unlike Corey and Ryan, Taylor wasn't thrilled with presents unless they involved adventure. One year in particular, when she was about ten years old, she unwrapped every gift without the slightest smile. I was disappointed at her reaction and told her so. She reciprocated with a note. "I am sorry I didn't acknowledge all the hard work you put into trying to make me happy, but that is not what Christmas is about for me. Thank you, Mommy, for taking me to midnight mass. It was the first time I was allowed to hold a candle in our dark church and sing." She added, "Going to midnight mass was the best gift I could have ever gotten. I have never felt that close to God. Thank you, Mommy." I am truly ashamed to write this: she understood what Christmas was all about, and I lost myself in a frenzy of shopping. Was she able to reach God on a deeper level than most?

Our long-standing traditions always started with making a gingerbread house, and this year was no exception. The girls kneaded gingerbread dough, sneaking scrumptious bites whenever possible while throwing it at each other. When it was time to build the house, we used melted Life Savers as glue, which acted more as an adornment than any kind of adhesive. Belly laughter erupted as the walls collapsed. "Okay, enough," I muttered. "This time, it is going to work!" In unison, the girls chuckled, "No, it's not." The more times the house fell apart, the happier they were.

When it was finally intact, I sat back and watched in delight as they covered the kitchen table with M&M's, jelly beans, candy canes, dots, and other confectionary delights. For just a moment, it felt as if life was normal again. However, Taylor's bald head popping around the table was stark reality. My mind wandered, *What if this is Taylor's last Christmas?* all the while forcing myself to keep a huge smile on my face. I quickly dispelled that thought and joined in fun.

Your mind works in odd ways when you have a very sick child. I learned a lifesaving lesson that worked for me throughout Taylor's illness: I strived to compartmentalize my thoughts. I embraced all the joy and happiness on the good days, and on the days Taylor was suffering or we were waiting for scan results, I allowed the extreme sadness and anxiety to take control, although I always tried my best to hide it from Taylor. This allowed me to achieve my greatest victory: allowing Taylor to live every moment she could, as if she were a regular kid.

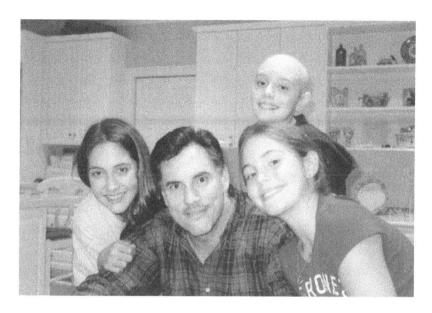

Taylor decided she wanted a Christmas tree for her room. She also had a secret agenda. Tales knew that I loved an all-white tree, but we alternated each year between white and colored to appease the kids. In my opinion, a color year, which happened to be this year, was a "tacky" year. Knowing Ryan had the creative gene in spades and the patience of a saint, Tales had her create an elegant, all-white tree for her room. "Look at my tree, Mommy," Taylor bellowed, as she unveiled it. "Do you love it?" Many a mother lives to make her child happy, but mine lived equally to make me smile. One nod of approval from me melted away all the problems of the world. At bedtime, I left the tree lit and watched Taylor fall asleep looking like an angel, aglow with happiness against a backdrop of shimmering white lights.

When Andrea's plane touched down at LaGuardia Airport, she and her family literally started running, trying to get to us as quickly as possible. Andrea knew a visit with their then two-year-old cousin, Samantha, and Uncle Bill meant the world to all three of my children. My kids, who were between the ages of two and seven the first time they met Uncle Bill, were absolutely smitten from the start with the strong, handsome, blond-haired, blue-eyed "Billy Boy," as they liked to call him. Actually, I think it was me who saddled Bill with that demeaning *nom de guerre*, and the name has lived on to this day. It takes a big man to settle into such a name, or at least one with a sense of humor! Bill has never complained.

When we first met him, Ryan giggled and stared at him; Corey was petrified of him; and Taylor took one look at him and knew she had a playmate for life. She absolutely adored him, and from that day forward, the two of them would roughhouse and play games endlessly when they were together.

When they arrived, the girls jumped for joy, picked Samantha up, embraced her, and spun her around in all her glory. She squealed, "Mewwy Christmas! I luff you!" Ryan put a big red bow atop Samantha's head, and Samantha fell on the floor in a puddle of laughter. Soon everyone was laughing so hard they could hardly breathe. No one was thinking about cancer.

We decided to continue our Christmas tree tradition of traveling over an hour into the wilderness to Jones Tree Farm, just so we could tramp up and down the hills through the cold, find a tree at the farthest point from the car, cut it down, drag it back, tie it to the roof, and drive it home—all for 20 percent more money than the perfectly formed tree down the street at the local nursery. What a plan!

Sammie, being so little, still had that stiff Frankenstein walk, especially since we bundled her in so many layers; the poor child could hardly move. "This tree is so niiiiiiice!" she giggled, running in and out of the dozens of trees, squealing. "No, Sammie," explained Tales. "We have to keep looking for the *perfect* tree." Soon Tales, looking like she was a member of the Taliban wrapped in her three scarves, fell behind. Heart wounded, I asked, "Are you okay, Tales? Do you need to turn back?" Taylor glared at me like I was a naughty child and then smiled and kept walking. She might've slowed down, but the hop in her step never dissipated.

As a young child, Taylor could never sit still. Even after a play date or school activity and homework, we had a lot of night left, and she needed to keep active. Many times, I told her, "Go outside and run laps around the house." She would run and run to exhaustion, panting with a big smirk and little puffy cheeks. She was nothing if not "all in" all the time.

We continued to celebrate the season until cancer got in our way, big time. Taylor was due for one more round of chemotherapy before the holiday. Taylor's oncologists disagreed as to which chemotherapy was best and asked us, behind each other's backs, to make the decision. So often parents are left with decisions about their child's treatment. Bob and I blindly made the choice before us with a very heavy heart. We prayed.

Sloan's rules required us to be in clinic by eight o'clock. If we missed the deadline, incriminating faces were quick to admonish us: "You are breaking our rules." Waking up a very sick child early and getting her out the door was not easily accomplished in a timely manner. In addition, I was fraught with guilt about leaving Ryan and Corey and truly outraged that, other than Andrea, no one in my family could or would help me. I was at least very blessed to have great friends who filled that void and came with us to the hospital time and time again.

So, each chemo morning, after I turned on the car and heated the seats, Bob would carry Taylor to the car, wrapped in blankets, and place her inside. He would send us off, saying, "You're not going for chemo. You are going to kill cancer; kick butt!" When she could muster the energy, Taylor would open her eyes, try to smile, and go right back to sleep.

Taylor's Christmas chemotherapy was a five-day treatment scheduled for the week prior to Christmas. We now understood that being "scheduled" for treatment was a far cry from actually receiving it. After several rounds of chemotherapy, your body's blood counts naturally decline. With each round, the body takes longer to recover. Blood counts need to be at a certain level to endure the next round of chemotherapy.

"Your platelets are way below acceptable limits to administer chemo," said Dr. Oscar in his stentorian voice, adding flippantly, "See you next week, Taylor." Another rule at Sloan: if your blood work was not acceptable on a Monday, you had to wait a whole week to try again. Taylor's eyes became red and swollen. I dug my eyes into his and hollered, "That is unacceptable, Dr. Oscar! Next week is Christmas." He glared back at me, indicating "too bad," as he callously turned his back and walked out.

This was going to be a big week of breaking rules. Doing things our way was the only way we had control and the only way to survive the medical system. I whispered, "Taylor, don't worry; I have a plan. You will not be in the hospital during Christmas." Her mischievous eyes sparkled with anticipation.

As we waited for the elevators, Taylor implored, "Tell me, Mommy; tell me!" I replied, "Just be patient. I will tell you as soon as we leave the building." Taylor melted in my arms, sporting a huge grin.

"Okay, Tales. Mommy is going to get into a lot of trouble, but we are going to White Plains Hospital (our local hospital) for blood counts. We will go every day until your platelets come up. They will come up in a few days, and then Scrooge, Dr. Oscar, will just have to administer chemo mid-week."

Taylor's eyes glazed over. Clearly the plan was not what she had expected. "But, Mommy, you know he won't do that."

"Oh, yes he will, my little T. I promise; you will be home for Christmas."

Two days later, Taylor's platelet count was rising. We decided to celebrate by going to her favorite restaurant, the Gasho House, a greasy, hibachi-style Japanese restaurant where the smells of soy sauce and stir-fry permeate your senses, not to mention your hair—not exactly a place up my alley. But Taylor loved watching them cook, and for a reason beyond my comprehension, she loved the food.

My flip phone rang. I looked at the number and showed it to Taylor. It was her nurse, Karen, who was quick to anger when things weren't done her way. Taylor's eyes grew wide with anticipation. "Okay, here we go, Tales!" I laughed.

With shrill exasperation, Karen screamed, "What do you think you're doing?" She was shouting so loudly, I had to quickly gesture toward Taylor to quell her laughter. Knowing it would irritate her further, I answered in a sing-songy, calm voice, "What did I do wrong, Karen?"

"How dare you go behind Dr. Oscar's back and get local blood counts?"

I replied innocently, "Oh, sorry, I didn't think White Plains Hospital would send Sloan the results."

Of course, I knew our local hospital always faxed Taylor's results to Sloan, and Karen knew I was no idiot. I continued, "Karen, Dr. Oscar is being unreasonable, considering it's Christmas. See you in clinic in a day or so when Taylor's platelet count is high enough."

Karen replied scathingly, "Sue! Don't you dare do this again or come to clinic. I will see you on *Monday*." At this point, Taylor and I couldn't stop giggling, as this irate woman continued to scream at me. Now she could hear us laughing.

A day or so later, when Taylor's platelets rose to an acceptable level, we arrived in the clinic unannounced. Karen refused to acknowledge us. Did she forget that we were dealing with a very sick twelve-year-old, whose only wish was to get chemotherapy so she could wake up Christmas morning in her own bed? Dr. Oscar came to see us, threw up his arms like a monkey, and said, "You are cleared. Start chemotherapy." Two points for Gryffindor!

After five straight days of intense chemotherapy, Taylor was ravaged and had lost her Christmas spirit. I drove home silently weeping while she slept. In years past, our house would've been aglow inside with decorations, gifts, glitter, and bows, and the outside would have been a mini winter wonderland, with majestic white lights, garland, wreaths, and candles shimmering against the backdrop of glistening, snow-covered trees. Andrea and I especially loved it because, as kids, we had always longed for beautiful outside Christmas lights. Our neighbors had an incandescent Rudolph, the envy of every child on the block, and at best, our dad would begrudgingly scatter one strand of lights upon a lonely bush outside our house. Whatever the reason, our family left no stone unturned when it came to Christmas décor. But this year our house was dim and forlorn, a sorrowful illustration of our family's state of mind and lack of bandwidth.

I had no idea that Bill and Andrea had decided to do something, anything, to cheer up the girls. While Tales and I were at the hospital, they hatched a plan to decorate the house from tip to toe before we returned home. "We can't have them come home to a dark house," said Andrea to the girls. "Get Uncle Bill; we're going shopping for lights and decorations." Bill was characteristically all in, willing to do anything in his power to help—yet another reason my girls adored him.

Knowing they only had a few hours until we returned, they grabbed the keys and quickly stormed out to buy Christmas lights and decorations. In a frenzy, they grabbed wreaths, bows, garland, and dozens of outdoor lights. It was all very exciting until they got home and realized that they, who had only been married a few short years, had never even gotten as far as Dad in the outdoor Christmas lighting department. They had no blazing idea what they were doing! Ryan and Corey looked dumbstruck, as they were used to parents who were veterans in this regard. Somehow, they found a way to jerry-rig the lights to frame the doorway and front porch. Bill was hanging by a thread on a ladder, sweat pouring down his cheeks in the dead of winter, while Samantha ran amuck in the snow on the front lawn, making snow angels and possibly eating yellow snow—no one will ever know.

As we turned the corner onto our street, I was dumbstruck. I shook Taylor awake. She arose from her slumped position and screamed with exhilaration, "Look, Mommy, at our house!" Andrea told me later, "We felt very proud, actually privileged, to be able to do even the slightest thing to make our sweet angel happy." They succeeded.

While all the Christmas festivities were going on, Bob was speaking to doctors all over the country in search of a creative, no-holds-barred approach. He read original research from dozens of doctors worldwide. He consulted with doctors at Children's Hospital of Philadelphia; St. Jude's; John's Hopkins; University of California, San Francisco; Mayo Clinic; Dana Farber; MD Anderson; and University of Michigan, amongst others. He kept hearing of new and different approaches, but our doctors at Sloan refused to consider any of them. Yet Taylor was showing signs of potentially serious side effects from her current treatment, and her spine was curving from her first surgery, causing additional pain and pulmonary risk. Her undefeatable little body was starting to cave in.

One icy, steel-grey morning, just before Christmas, Bob's nightmares were confirmed when he met with Taylor's doctors. Dr. Oscar, nonplussed, said, "She's not responding well to treatment. Let's finish the prescribed eighteen rounds of high-dose chemo and take it from there." I'm not sure if Dr. Oscar said it or not, but Bob understood him to mean that we should continue giving Taylor chemotherapy that he knew wasn't working, and if and when it didn't work, he would consider experimental treatments. We believe Dr. Oscar's rigid determination to have Taylor finish standard protocol until she failed was part of his adherence to precise and rigid treatment protocols shared by all the major hospitals to create reliable research databases—but it was at Taylor's expense.

Disturbed, Bob called me and said, "It's time to challenge them to think outside the box!" It was time for her doctors to come up with new and innovative treatments in place of the ones she was getting. Taylor, in her typical style, had already made that clear when she paraded into clinic sporting her "Think Outside the Box" T-shirt for giggles. However, my favorite was "Bad Hair Day," which she wore when she was bald.

Fighting cancer means asking questions and questioning the answers. Questioning should never cease, no matter how comfortable you are with your doctors and your treatment plan. Parents desperately want to believe their doctors are gods who can cure everything. We learned to ask detailed questions, putting the doctors on the spot so they couldn't wiggle their way out.

We were finding quickly that opinions on treatment varied enormously. Had we sat blindly and refrained from forcibly asking questions, getting second opinions, and sometimes breaking the rules, no one would have done it for us. We were Taylor's only true advocates. With certainty, I can say that Bob's tenacious ability to never stop researching and speaking to doctors across the world extended Taylor's life dramatically. Knowledge is *power*!

A Hope Renewed

It was time to make our move. Fortunately, one of my best friends, Donna, with her striking blue eyes and beautiful thick reddish hair, whom Taylor adored, personally knew the head of pediatric surgery at Columbia. As a courtesy to Donna, Dr. Altman, a brusque and autocratic chief who had the intimidating demeanor of a grizzled veteran of accomplishment, agreed to see Bob on Christmas Eve at half past one.

After listening to Bob tell our story, Dr. Altman recommended we see Dr. Jim Garvin, who was, at the time, heading up hematology/oncology and stem cell transplant. We had read the bios on all of the doctors on the pediatric oncology unit. Dr. Garvin seemed a strange choice given that his most impressive accomplishments seemed to have been in pediatric brain tumors.

Bob asked Dr. Altman, "Why aren't we seeing the department's osteosarcoma expert?" Altman's reaction must have been practiced repeatedly during his more than thirty years of reducing aspiring surgical fellows to Jell-O. The glasses came off. He turned from his computer to look Bob in the eye and asked very bluntly, "Mr. Matthews, am I making this referral, or are you?"

This was not a rhetorical question. While he waited for Bob to answer, Dr. Altman turned back to his computer, where he made some notes, sent an email, and looked up some information. When he turned back, he seemed prepared to answer Bob's apparently insolent question.

"I don't know why your daughter hasn't reacted to the standard treatments. Apparently, they don't know at Sloan either. Dr. Garvin is the smartest physician I know and does more reading and research than anyone I know. That is who I would go to for solving the intractable." With that he stood, gestured to Bob to follow, and walked him through the labyrinthine hallways to pediatric oncology where he handed Bob off to Dr. Garvin personally. It was apparent that the surgical fellows weren't the only ones intimidated by Dr. Altman. Dr. Garvin reacted as though he were addressing a superior officer.

Bob had arrived with scans under his arm and pages upon pages of history and personal research. We had learned, after a wasted trip to the renowned hospital Dana Farber, to always bring copies of the scans. It is essential to maintain all records yourself.

The clinic was empty except for Bob, Dr. Garvin, a couple of nurses cleaning up the last details before the holiday, and a few patients who were being admitted. Everyone else had gone home for the holiday. Bob had no idea what to expect, but instead of a cursory consultation, he had an in-depth discussion with Dr. Garvin, a brilliant, calm, and kindhearted doctor whose compassion shined through his ocean-blue eyes. They discussed Taylor's history, including Bob's entire ongoing search for creative additions to her protocols, our concerns about what the scans said, and what to do next.

Dr. Garvin involved colleagues from the research lab, clinic, and pathology who wandered in and out of the conversation. Hours passed, and still he was asking endless questions. Bob asked whether he thought he could help and what ideas he had about a change in protocol. Dr. Garvin was modest in his response, but he suggested that he could help. To Bob's amazement, Dr. Garvin was already using some of the medicines Bob was looking for and was completely open to anything else within reason that could help turn the tide for Tales. He had unique ideas and was willing to start from scratch and look for creative approaches. He was willing to take the case.

Bob knew that we had just raised our chances. That meeting resulted in a complete, outside-the-box, stretch-the-envelope approach that ended up making all the difference. Although Bob knew nothing more than he had known when he first went in, he at least knew Dr. Garvin was going to think creatively, and he wasn't going to preach about finishing the standard protocols to protect the research database for the Children's Oncology Group.

When the phone finally rang, my heart skipped a beat. I wasn't sure what to expect. "I am going to be late for Christmas Eve dinner. I am still with Dr. Garvin, and he has many ideas!" Bob exclaimed. I could hear the relief and sense of accomplishment in his voice. In a matter of hours, Taylor's prognosis had turned from exceedingly grim to exceedingly hopeful. Two different doctors, two different hospitals, and the make-it-or-break-it treatment plan affecting the life of our twelve-year-old child went from one end of the spectrum to the other: one full of sorrow, the other full of hope. It turned out to be our best Christmas ever.

Dr. Garvin got to the point quickly and showed enthusiasm for Bob's ideas. Taylor had been on the standard secondary protocol for osteosarcoma ever since the standard primary protocol had failed, a position that Dr. Oscar would never accept, even though Taylor's scans showed no shrinkage and even possible growth, and Taylor's tumors removed during surgery showed minimal narcosis (death of cancer cells). More treatments of the same kind were a poor bet and possibly a waste of precious time or, worse, harmful to Taylor. Dr. Garvin recommended two new chemotherapies in combination. We learned that a combination of two chemotherapies is very common; the idea is to hit the tumor in two different ways simultaneously, without overlapping toxicities to the patient.

The chemotherapies Dr. Garvin suggested struck Bob as odd based upon all his research. Bob pushed him to explain, knowing that doctors are not accustomed to being questioned. But instead of the imperious or dismissive response he was expecting, Bob got a deep explanation of the chemical differences and possible differences in the mechanism of the chemotherapies he chose. After studying Taylor's cancer and her reactions to the drugs, Dr. Garvin thought this approach might be more effective. "We'll know pretty quickly if it's working," Garvin said. "Let's see how the scans look after a full cycle." Of course, Bob continued to pepper him with questions. Garvin patiently answered every one.

By late January 2004, we had officially moved hospitals, and Taylor was now a hundred blocks up the street at Columbia. On our first day there, we sat alone on an old, leather circular couch with our feet planted firmly on a faded multi-colored floor, if only for balance. By now, we were used to a pediatric cancer clinic but everything and everyone looked different. We were still prisoners of cancer jail, just in a different place. I was still a veteran "cancer mom," a title I will forever hold, belonging to a club in which no one ever wants to be a member.

Although a lot changed at Columbia, one thing remained the same: "Mommyyyyyy, I am so bored, and I miss my friends!"

"I know, sweetheart," I offered. "And I know it isn't the same, but I'm here for you, no matter what." She frowned. She wanted people her own age! Taylor had made a few good friends at Sloan, but even that had its problems. I remember Taylor saying, "Mommy, I don't want to make any new friends in the hospital anymore; they all die." I had no answer.

At this point in our journey, we had to separate from everyone at Sloan and establish a confidence level with our new caregivers at Columbia. It was like she had switched schools in the middle of the year. We didn't know Columbia's procedures, the staff members' personalities, or how far we could push them.

An oncologist named Dr. Jessie Carson greeted us warmly. She was a feisty, tiny woman with a brilliant mind and five children of her own. Taylor grew to love her. Dr. Carson introduced us to our new nurse practitioner, Jane, a tall woman with short strawberry-blonde hair, a heart that stretched a mile wide, and a passion for Bruce Springsteen. Then we met our primary nurse, Karen, who always wore brightly colored scrubs and a matching smile, and whose compassion and love for Taylor shone as bright as the sun. Jane and Karen became a part of our family.

Taylor had a sweet spot for her new oncologist, Dr. Garvin, whose gentle bedside manner, punctuated by his small, rounded spectacles and bow tie, made her comfortable. Each day the group greeted us with huge smiles and can-do attitudes. It was extremely important for Taylor to trust her nurses and doctors and feel at ease in her new surroundings, and she did.

We soon met Christine, a beautiful woman, tall and thin, with black, lustrous hair and a warm smile. Christine, an alternative medicine therapist, never tired of helping children with cancer and had a soft spot for Taylor. Taylor adored her right back. Not only was she hilarious, but Christine always, and I mean *always,* had a story to tell. In time, Christine's role would prove essential.

The Love of Family

A few years earlier, for my fortieth birthday, Bob surprised me with a trip to France. Andrea and Bill, who were engaged at the time, flew up from Charlotte to babysit. They didn't know what they were in for with our three young girls. The kids were psyched!

We left Andrea and Bill a to-do list for the week. Taylor, of course, had her own items to add. Andrea can't fully recall the long list of ailments and activities that Taylor recited because they were overshadowed by her final statement: "*And,*" she said, pausing for added emphasis, "my butt *always* itches!" Andrea can't help laughing every time she retells the story. "It was a very appropriate comment," says Andrea, "because Taylor always was a pain in the butt!"

Before that trip to France, Bob and I had never traveled without our kids, so this was a big break in protocol. I knew Andrea and Bill were the best babysitters the kids could dream of, and for Tales, that meant extra time with her favorite guy, Uncle Billy Boy. They played games together all week, with the *denouement* being a trip to Sports Time, a place that, at the time, had over one hundred and fifty arcade games and laser tag.

After Bob and I had spent three days alone in Nice, Andrea, Bill, and the girls flew to Paris, where we all met for the remainder of the trip. Upon their arrival in Paris, everyone seemed a little tired, but no one more than Andrea and Bill, who looked shell-shocked after spending three days taking care of three kids. It was hilarious. They had gone from zero to one hundred in a flat minute and were glad to have made it out alive.

We asked the girls if they had fun, and they all said yes—except Taylor, of course, who had to comment, "Well, Shommy," which was her nickname of choice for me at the time, "it was fun but Aunt Annie didn't make my bed all week." Busted! Such a little beast! All in all, the trip was a huge success. Together we literally danced in the streets of Paris and in the subway cars, bellowing tunes from an old Italian Lou Monte record my mother used to play for us, recited silly poems about Speedy Gonzalez ("the fastest mouse in all of Mexico"), ate, drank wine, and laughed until our bellies hurt.

When we finally had a week off from the hospital, it wasn't surprising that the only place Taylor dreamed of going was to visit Andrea, Bill, and Samantha in North Carolina. As much as we wanted to fulfill her dreams, Taylor still had a weakened immune system, so she couldn't fly on a commercial flight. We weren't taking no for an answer very well, but it all seemed hopeless until somehow Bill convinced a business acquaintance to fly her to North Carolina on his private jet—no easy feat. Taylor was overjoyed; her face beamed with excitement.

When the time came, Taylor and I were alone in the plane with the pilot and co-pilot. We cuddled together, looking out at the open, clear, blue sky. It was a magical moment for Taylor, one of total freedom. Wrapped up in the joy of seeing Taylor so happy, I embraced her, but I couldn't help thinking that the sky and its beauty were the closest analogy I knew to heaven, and that someday Taylor could be in this unknown place. I wept inside, hoping and praying that I would never see that day arrive.

While in Charlotte, Taylor suddenly and abruptly began vomiting. "Mommy, I'm so weak," she whispered, laying in Andrea's family room watching television. I knew I had to get her to bed immediately. Just then, Uncle Bill came around the bend and scooped Tales up in his arms, carrying her up the stairs to the guest room. "I got you, Tales," he told her gently, deep compassion blinding his heartsick eyes. I tucked myself in next to my baby girl, and as we lay in bed together like two teddy bears, Taylor said to me, "Mommy, Uncle Bill really loves me." Tales and Uncle Bill had always had a strong bond, but this sealed their hearts forever.

Go Big or Go Home!

Columbia encouraged us to contact the Make a Wish Foundation. Taylor, always one to think outside the box and push her boundaries, "wished" for a tree house in our backyard, complete with a hole in the roof for a telescope to see the star that the Onoratos, our dear family friends, had registered in her name. One of Taylor's passions was climbing trees, but beyond her love for trees, this wish seemed completely out of the blue. Years later she confided in Bob and me,

"What I really wanted was a pool, but I thought Daddy would say no." It haunts Bob to this day. In retrospect, building a pool, which we eventually did a few years later at Taylor's insistence, was far easier.

Taylor's excitement grew as the date of her Make a Wish appointment approached. She was neutropenic, which meant she was not allowed to leave the house for fear of germs. "Mommy, pleeeease can we go to Barnes & Noble to get tree house books? I want to be able to show them what I want!" Goosebumps covered my body as I remembered years past when I regularly took all my girls to Barnes & Noble. Those were the days when the four of us would sit on the floor, constantly moving between rows, combing the aisles for books each of them wanted to read. Ryan's favorite was *Nancy Drew*, and Corey loved *The Royal Diaries*. Unable to say no, I replied, "Okay, Tales, but you need to wear your heavy blue coat," as if the heavier it was, the more germ resistant it would be, "your red, green, and white striped scarf that you can wrap around your face several times, your favorite pink hat, and a surgical mask over your face." Taylor immediately obliged. I grimaced as I saw her emerge, with only her piercing brown eyes visible through her kooky outfit, but it didn't seem to faze her. No matter what she looked like, her goal was to go!

We spent over an hour scouring tree house books. I can still hear her giggle as she turned the pages, finding one outrageous tree house picture after another. She seemed to be dreaming of the Swiss Family Robinson house, similar to the one in Disney World. Clearly, she had forgotten that the Robinson family was trying to build an *actual* new house after their ship was stranded off the coast of an island. But, like the Robinsons, who lost their way after being besieged by pirates, Taylor, besieged by cancer, was stranded off course and was determined to rebuild.

Together our family chose the biggest and oldest tree in our yard on which to build the tree house. However, late the following week, Mother Nature intervened with an enormous windstorm. The chosen tree fell, crushing our trampoline, the neighbor's fence, and Taylor's plans. You can't make this up. We had been living in our home for over ten years, and just then the tree decided to keel over.

We immediately started working on Plan B. No tree in our yard could possibly support the tree house that Taylor had in mind, anyway, so we built the tree house around a new tree that we planted. In the end, it was equipped with six bunk beds (outfitted in Pottery Barn Kids' bedding in a rainbow of colors), a loft, a wrap-around deck, windows with shutters to match our house, baseboard heating, electricity, and an alarm, so I could feel everyone sleeping over would be safe at night. London has the London Eye. We affectionately named Taylor's creation the "Edgemont Eyesore." Taylor's final product had little relation to a tree house. It was more like a second home and was definitely a bit over the top for the Make a Wish folks. They understandably bowed out gracefully, still leaving Taylor with one wish.

Answered Prayers

After Taylor's first dose of the highly toxic chemotherapy prescribed as part of Dr. Garvin's new protocol, she was debilitated and emotionally distraught. I remember walking down the hospital corridor feeling like I was sinking in quicksand. Just then, Dr. Carson came running toward me like she had just won the lottery. She embraced me, joyously screaming, "Sue! Taylor's tumors show significant shrinkage, and several tumors are dead!" Her luminous blue eyes were like reflecting pools beaming sunlight, warming me from the inside out. A rush of adrenaline and joy pulsed through my veins, followed by a calmness and serenity I never knew existed.

After the second cycle, Taylor was in remission. The only problem was, as Dr. Garvin compassionately explained to Taylor, "Even though you're in remission, you need one more dose of chemotherapy to make sure every cancer cell is killed." Without hesitation, Taylor agreed, trusting everything Dr. Garvin suggested. However, the red warning lights, indicating danger zone, were blinking, and we all knew it. Taylor's body could take little more. Her doctors feared her immune system would not return for weeks after this last round of chemotherapy, leaving her in a very precarious situation, perilously open to infection. There is a limit to how much of this poison a body can take.

I thought, *How can this be?* Her life has been saved, and now the chemo could kill her? Dr. Garvin, always a step ahead of us, told me, "Sue, a stem cell rescue would most likely bring her immune system back in a week." My body slumped forward. I rubbed my eyes, and I almost cried with relief. Luckily, in his quest for second opinions, just a few months after Taylor's initial diagnosis, Bob had been told by Johns Hopkins to harvest Taylor's stem cells for potential use in the future. Taylor's doctors at Sloan fought us about harvesting Taylor's cells, most likely because, as we found out years later, they never really thought Tales would make it that far. Yet, we insisted.

Harvesting cells is accomplished by inserting a stent, a ten-minute procedure requiring very little anesthesia. Back when we arrived at Sloan on the day of the procedure, however, the always-adversarial Dr. Oscar turned to Taylor and said, "Sorry, we don't have an anesthesiologist available." He was annoyed, I assume, because the procedure hadn't been his idea. Taylor hissed, "Fine, I will do the procedure without anesthesia!"

When you let her down, made a mistake, or missed a promise, she let you have it right between the eyes, in a withering sort of way—much like a Marine drill sergeant but with fewer (and more acceptable) words. She had resilience and fortitude. With an exasperated sigh, Dr. Oscar turned his back on us, not wanting us to see his blazing red face, tapped on his computer for a few minutes, and finally said, "Fine. I found an anesthesiologist. Wait outside for a few minutes, and we will be set to go." Slam-dunk! Nothing or no one was standing in our way.

Now, at Columbia, giving Taylor back her stem cells by IV would be a fifteen-minute process. The only side effect was a bad taste and a horrible smell of sulfur. When the procedure was complete, they stuck half an orange in her mouth, and that was it.

The procedure worked just as hoped. Within two weeks, Tales had her immune system back, weeks sooner than she would have without her stem cell rescue.

Bob recalls his conversation with Dr. Garvin as a typically low-key recitation of the facts, but it was clear there was news to report: "After three cycles, the radiology report suggests there is no evidence of live tumors in her chest, and the tumors in her leg could not be found on the scan!" Bob couldn't believe his ears! Gone? Dormant? Dead tumors? You can't imagine the joy that flooded his heart.

In a quiet moment several weeks later, Bob asked Dr. Garvin why he selected the chemotherapies he did when they weren't traditionally prescribed for osteosarcoma, and why he felt so strongly they might work. He advised Bob that he had gone back to Sloan to review Taylor's tumor and spoke with the pathologist. The pathologist remembered getting the sample from the surgery/oncology group with a statement that her cancer was osteosarcoma. The pathologist confirmed osteosarcoma, but I believe he commented that it was always a strange sample. It didn't look like normal osteosarcoma and wasn't as structured or well-formed in organization like it should have been. It was sloppy. In fact, he continued, it almost resembled a soft-tissue sarcoma.

That was all Garvin needed to hear. If it looks like a duck and quacks like a duck, treat it like a duck. And so, Taylor was given a chemotherapy regimen more commonly used for soft-tissue sarcomas. One doctor, determined to ask more questions rather than presuming he knew the answers, had led Taylor into remission.

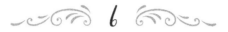

Ĭ Will Survive

Cancer may have started the fight, but I will finish it.

–The Fresh Quotes

A Return to Normalcy

Throughout treatment, Taylor had pleaded, "I just want to be normal." Now that Taylor was in remission, the truth was, normal life had become alien. Returning to normalcy wasn't as easy as we thought it would be.

Tales and I took a simple trip to the mall, a place we had frequented so often throughout her childhood. The bright lights, the colorful clothing hanging in the windows, and the aroma of dough pretzels and Starbucks coffee deluged us. Most striking were the faces of people seeming to be living without a care in the world. I couldn't remember ever feeling that way. We had become accustomed to our safety zone of the hospital, even with all its ugliness. Neither of us anticipated how difficult it would be to navigate this, a maze of conventional circumstances and places. The battle had ceased, but we were still in the war zone.

Acclimating to normal life was excruciating. Fitting in with a gaggle of drama-filled teenage girls is not an easy feat, even in the best of circumstances, but try doing it in Taylor's shoes. Before diagnosis, she had been in elementary school, when fashion, boys, and boobs were not part of normal conversations. She had been a robust, cherubic tween with skinned knees and chubby cheeks. When she returned, she was a frail thirteen-year-old with short, frizzy chemo hair and too many scars to count. Her friends had started to develop, and they all had the same long, perfectly styled hair flowing down their backs. She had missed out on most of junior high and was no longer easily accepted. Taylor was lost but determined.

I found her in the living room one night, boiling over with anger, tears brimming in her eyes. "Mommy, they left me out. I was not invited to one of the biggest 'cool' parties." I tried to reply, but she stopped me, spitting out words rapid fire and ending with, "I am going. I will somehow get invited." And she did.

Taylor was relentless and eventually succeeded in re-acclimating, but at an enormous emotional strain and cost to her self-esteem. Her emotional scars were far deeper than her actual ones, and although she appeared strong on the outside, even a small scratch could unseal her wounds, causing her to hemorrhage salty tears.

I Did It My Way

The after-effects of Taylor's very first surgery, when the doctors removed her primary tumor without putting in a prosthesis to close the space left behind in her rib cage, were in full bloom now. Taylor's spine had moved into that empty space, resulting in severe scoliosis and tremendous pain. Her head was so tilted, it practically rested on one shoulder. Nevertheless, her doctors at Columbia did not support surgery to realign her spine. We refused their reasoning and were unwilling to accept their answer. Our experience with resistance at Sloan about harvesting Taylor's stem cells, which likely ended up saving her life, was too fresh in our minds.

After many sleepless nights and fruitless consultations, we realized it was time to take matters into our own hands. In the summer of 2004, we decided to push ahead with scoliosis surgery to give Taylor control over her body. Taylor's orthopedic surgeon at Columbia, Dr. David Roye (or as we called him, Dr.

David) was one of the true stars of Taylor's journey. He was a gifted and aggressive advocate as a surgeon, as well as an incredibly caring and attentive person. We would also find out later that he is one of the country's most respected pediatric orthopedic surgeons. He was ready and willing to take on the challenge of repairing Taylor.

Taylor came through the surgery beautifully and with 100 percent correction! Dr. David understood that he was treating a child, not a cancer patient, and that quality of life mattered. Years later, I saw Dr. David at a fundraiser and reminded him of his heroic contribution. He laughed. "Mrs. Matthews, there have only been three times in my career where I was truly scared in a surgery. That was one of them. But I couldn't deny her a chance."

Taylor endured an enormous amount of pain following the scoliosis surgery, but there was no question in her mind that it was worth it. Most of her oncologists remained stunned that we had elected to subject Taylor to so much suffering. To needle the doctors who had not supported her surgery, I decided to pull a "Taylor" stunt. She was famous for her pajamas covered in funny sayings, such as "Boys Are Smelly," "It's All About Me," and, our personal favorite, "This Sucks." I thought the "This Sucks" pair, which I of course owned as well, was particularly appropriate attire for me in the ICU after surgery. Try to imagine me, a middle-aged mom, braless, in that outfit. Somehow thumbing my nose at the world gave me great satisfaction.

It didn't take Taylor long to regain her sense of adventure and her deep-seated need to always seek out fun. Two weeks post-surgery, while en route to pick up Ryan and Corey from camp in the Adirondacks, Taylor asked, "Can I go waterskiing?" I turned around and said, "You are crazy! The Steri-Strips are still on from surgery. I am not calling Dr. David, but you can." With that, she picked up her phone, and to our surprise, he said yes! Again, Dr. David knew the importance of letting Taylor live her life to the fullest and on her terms. She waterskied like a champ.

One time, in clinic, Taylor received cupping therapy to relieve the pain in her shoulders caused by her first two thoracotomies. Cupping therapy involves lifting the skin through suction cups, bringing blood to the surface and improving circulation. At this point, Taylor was a seasoned veteran of the clinic. She approached Karen, whose calming personality always assuaged our nerves, and yelled in a high-pitched voice, "My back is red and bruised!" While examining Taylor, Karen's eyes met mine with grave concern.

When a child with cancer is bruising, it can mean many things. It might simply mean the child needs a platelet transfusion, or it could be a sign of leukemia, a possible side effect of high-dose chemotherapy. All I could do was put my head down and try desperately to hold in my tears of laughter. Karen immediately said, "I'm paging the doctor." I didn't say a word, leaving Taylor in charge. Fortunately, Taylor knew she had crossed the line when Karen's demeanor changed, and said, giggling, "Got you, Karen!" Karen's expression was not a happy one, but she, too, understood Taylor's need to relieve tension and still be a child.

Ride for the Roses

A colleague of Bob's had introduced us to the Lance Armstrong Foundation. One of their representatives asked Taylor if she would like to participate in the "Ride for the Roses," a long-standing biking event that Lance created after he won his battle with cancer. Her answer was abundantly clear from the quiet little smile that beamed from her cherry-red lips. Needless to say, we were all thrilled.

As the sun rose over Austin, Texas, thousands of cyclists saddled up. The clanking of bikes hummed in the background. The excitement in the air was palpable. We were among thousands of people, most of whom donned the newly famous Livestrong yellow wristbands and all of whom were in Austin for the same reason: to present a united front of survivors, patients, and families battling against the demon of cancer.

This was not as much a race as a crusade of endurance. The fight to cross the finish line symbolized the fight for survival for so many cancer warriors. No one wants to join the "cancer club," but here, at this moment, the comfort and camaraderie of this group felt like a warm blanket covering shivering shoulders. It felt healing. Our hands were bound, our mouths gagged by an insidious serpent, but the ride freed us, if only for a moment, to do something, anything, to break out of its grasp. Even more than healing in the moment, it represented hope for the future.

We were handed five racing bibs with the words "I Am a Survivor" printed in black against a "Lance Armstrong yellow" background. As I fastened mine to my shirt, my heart beat rapidly with profound joy. Taylor now belonged to the group called "survivors." Always the one to get the troops going, Bob called out, "Are we ready?" We all nodded wordlessly. Bob alone sported a huge grin; the rest of us were stoic. We didn't know what to think.

We rode like the wind, actually kind of like the breeze, until we hit mile three, where we encountered a very steep hill. Taylor was ahead of me, now struggling with each pedal. All I could see was her black helmet and her Livestrong T-shirt on her very thin frame. I could not see the expression on her face, but I imagine she was gritting her teeth as she strained to make it up the vertical incline. I felt the same anxiety I did many years before, following her as she skied down her first black diamond run. I yelled ahead to her, "Let's just walk it." She barely turned her head and kept on riding. Bob, Ryan, and Corey were already at the top of the hill watching us, Bob with a smirk on his face, knowing Taylor was not going to give up. She made it to the top of the hill and quickly pushed forward, not wanting any applause or recognition.

At the split in road, we turned toward the long route, and for the first few miles, we rode with Lance and about seven thousand of his closest friends. We never actually saw him, but truth be told, he wasn't the highlight.

Toward the end of the course, we rode down a long lane past a grandstand filled with a boisterous, cheering crowd. As we got to the last quarter mile, the road separated. Survivors were directed to the right and all others to the left. Tales looked at me sheepishly as I pointed with a very firm expression on my face, telling her to pedal down the survivorship lane. She peeled off by herself and biked the last part alone, struggling to finish. There were no other survivors for hundreds of yards.

As she crossed the finish line, the crowd erupted into wild cheering, and her name boomed from a loudspeaker. It could have been the Olympic gold medal finish of the five-thousand-meter race. She was handed a single yellow rose and had her picture taken. She was spent, barely able to smile for the camera, but her eyes radiated with pride. The fact that a rose is a universal symbol of love was not lost on us. It was one of those moments when all the stars aligned, pure happiness felt tangible, and our hearts pounded together, swelling with joy.

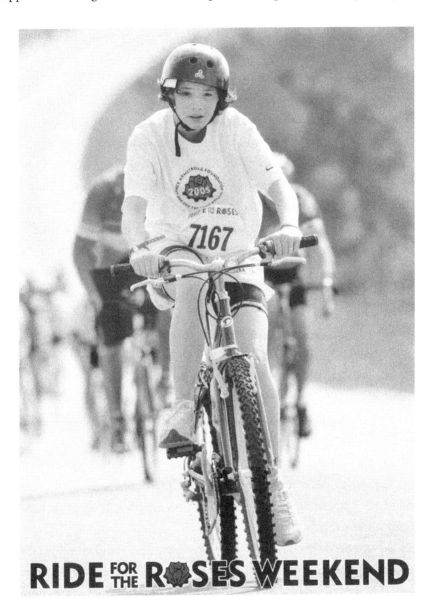

Comfort in Traditions

That fall, I was determined to resume a favorite Matthews family tradition: our annual wine party. Ten years prior, I couldn't have known that purchasing Bob a winemaking book on a whim would turn into so much fun. Back in the day, the book piqued my interest simply because it reminded me of the stories of my long-gone Italian grandfather who, in the 1940s, made wine in his bathtub in the Bronx, carrying on his family's traditions from Italy.

Grandpa's customs, straight from Rome, were now being carried on in our small town some fifty years later, with my Anglo-Saxon husband at the helm. At the time, one of Bob's favorite phrases was, "White wine is for *cooking*," and, therefore, we only considered making red. Wine gets its color from the grape's skin. So, of course, making red wine meant more fun and a bigger mess!

When the kids were little, my parents, Bob, the girls, and I endeavored to make our first bottle of wine. This involved crushing an enormous amount of grapes in a huge bucket (big enough to hold four to five adults)—with our feet! The scene was straight out of the iconic *I Love Lucy* episode, where Lucy hilariously finds herself wrestling with a crazy local Italian lady in a vat of grapes. In our bucket, instead of a wacky Lucille Ball and a fiery Italian woman, we had my mother Rita (equal parts Lucy and the crazy Italian lady), Ryan, Taylor, and two-year old Corey, a newly potty-trained toddler.

Being that my mom was always up for a good laugh, she agreed to get into the bucket with the girls. We were all laughing, having a grand old time, when Bob suddenly exclaimed, "Sue, with all that liquid Corey might pee in the wine!" He quickly scooped her up and out of the bucket, put her on the grass, and, sure enough, within seconds she peed. Our eyes all bulged out of our heads as we watched the scene unfold as she had come so close to ruining the wine. I'm not sure I've laughed that hard again since.

Afterwards, we fermented the wine, put it in oak barrels, and then bottled and corked it, just like the experts. Bob custom-designed the label with a picture of our three girls, and we aptly named the wine, *Les Filles de Matthews*. We gave the bottles to our friends, who, I'm certain, were more excited to see the label than drink the wine.

In the later years, we had invited our friends to help. The unsuspecting were shocked to discover they had actually been invited to de stem crates of grapes off their vines, sanitize their feet, and then literally get in a bucket and vigorously crush the grapes barefoot on our patio.

So on this day, as always, the moms stood by while the dads got into the larger bucket and the kids into the smaller bucket. In the end, everyone was drenched from top to toe, with grapes between their toes, in their hair, and soaking down their clothes, now permanently stained red.

As we once again handed out the bottles to our friends, it felt like life had circled its way back to those pre-cancer glory days.

The Lost Siblings

With Taylor in remission, Ryan and Corey were trying to start the school year with their own sense of normalcy—yet things were still far from normal. Having a sibling who has cancer is devastatingly complicated for the healthy children. They naturally felt forgotten as our family's focus and energy was on Taylor, yet they, too, shared the burden, fears, stress, and dislocation that came with the tragic turns of Taylor's journey. Life had become a rollercoaster, and they never knew when the next downhill plunge was approaching.

Although Ryan and Corey never verbally expressed jealousy or anger, it had to have been buried deep inside them. We tried so hard to impress upon them that they were not alone in their emotions, but because their problems seemed, at the time, so minute compared to Taylor's, many times they got swept under the rug.

Ryan, now fifteen, believed we had finally won and that Taylor was going to be fine, but things were still difficult. To some extent, she was still dreading going back to high school. Corey, now ten, was still struggling to find her place in the world. She was so tragically young when Taylor was diagnosed. She swung back and forth between fear, concern, guilt, frustration, confusion, and normal childhood angst. Returning to school showed her that—for better or for worse— the experience of Taylor's illness had changed her as a person, and she would do well to accept it.

As for me, I prayed the school year would start out well. It had been a long, hard road to get to a place that resembled anything close to normal, and I hoped Taylor's remission meant I could spend a lot of quality time with Corey and Ryan. Now that I had a moment to breathe, the realization of my sudden absence in their lives sliced my heart like a razor. From one day to the next, I had all but vanished. I'll never be able to turn back time and change the way our story unfolded. My heart aches that I was not present for them at their young ages. But I can only hope that, through it all, they always knew how much they were so truly loved.

Back to Biking

It had been only a few years since our final "pre-cancer" trip to London, but it seemed like a lifetime. With Taylor in remission, the idea of getting away together as a family was exhilarating. The girls nearly exploded with excitement when Bob and I suggested a biking trip for vacation. Prior to Taylor's diagnosis, some of our best trips were biking through Europe. This trip, only six months after our Lance Armstrong bike ride, seemed worlds apart. The Lance Armstrong trip was about cancer. This trip was a family celebration.

Naturally, we were worried about our choice; Taylor had lost about 30 percent of her lung capacity and a great deal of her strength, as evidenced by the Lance Armstrong event. However, she looked healthy, and she was fiercely determined to rebound and get her old self back. So, we left behind all our concerns about work, school, and health and headed to Normandy, France.

When we arrived, we met our very lovely tour guide, Angie, a young blonde who also had limited lung capacity due to her own battle with cancer. As a team, Taylor and Angie were unstoppable. Each morning we would awaken to a feeling of freedom and exuberance as we immersed ourselves in the local culture. Every ride, we took in our surroundings and reveled in the thrill of coasting along a great downhill. On our first day, Taylor's skinny legs pedaled furiously, trudging up the hills at only a quarter of the pace, leaving us at the back of the pack. I was apprehensive until I saw her face, which told a very different story. She was not going to give up or give in. As heartbreaking as it was to see Taylor "handicapped," the beauty of seeing her climbing up and down the hills of the

French countryside for three or four hours at a time, outside of a hospital, in the fresh air, and on vacation, is a sight that will stay with me forever.

The trip unfolded with great success, as several times Taylor and Angie made it to the top of the pack, and no matter where we biked, we appreciated the gift of Taylor's health. Our family back together again was a miracle, and we knew that even if it might be temporary, it was still happening, and we recognized it as a forever moment. As difficult as it was, our story had made us hyper-aware of all the wonderful things in our lives and forced us to savor them.

Aloha!

Our successful biking trip re-infected us with our long-lost friend, the "travel bug." We planned a trip to Kona, Hawaii. When the wheels hit the ground and the jumbo jet halted to a full stop, the smiles on my girls' faces lit up. As we departed the airport, it looked like we had landed on a barren planet. The sight of enormous, black boulders set against the azure-blue sky was stunning. I looked at the girls' mesmerized faces. No one spoke a word. Streaked on the black boulders in white chalk were messages of encouragement to the participants of the Ironman, a race held there every year. We were not there to watch the race, but the words welcomed us to the island just the same.

At our hotel, we encountered lush, green grass and inhaled the fragrant aroma of flowers budding in every color. Our suite overlooked the ocean, as well as a magnificent pond filled with rare species of fish. We later learned this pond was called King's Pond, carved out of natural lava and filled with 1.8 million gallons of fresh and ocean water. It contained over four-thousand tropical fish from ninety-eight species. As we swam with the exotic fish, my thoughts jumped from how blessed Bob and I were to share some of life's greatest experiences with our kids, to how we had endured the worst tragedy a family could face. Pre-cancer, I had always believed that life had no meaning without one's health and a heart filled with love. Now, I really understood that message, in full-blown bold.

One evening we ordered a picnic dinner under the stars. Seated at our beach table, we slipped off our shoes and let our bare feet sink into the soft white sand. The sun set in vivid, golden colors, marking the end of the day. After dinner, we were ushered to a place on the beach where a small fire, encircled with stones, was ablaze, its beautiful yellow and red flames illuminating our way. Just when we thought it couldn't get any better, the waiters came over with a huge tray of confectionary delights. "Look, they're bringing us chocolate, marshmallows, and graham crackers! I think we're going to make s'mores!" exclaimed Corey, bouncing up and down.

With filled bellies, we laid on our backs staring at the stars. It was now pitch dark on a clear night. The moon cast its light on the sea, the fire illuminated our faces, and the stars glowed from above. The sound of the waves echoed in the background, and the smell of the ocean and salty air enveloped our senses. In that moment, I felt caught between the beauty of heaven and earth. I saw myself floating above the crashing waves, staring down at my beautiful family, as I pleaded with God to keep us together as a family of five. I was in a state of panic, fearing Taylor would relapse; yet my surroundings couldn't have been more peaceful and serene.

We were all lost in our thoughts and didn't speak for a long time. I remember wishing I could hop into the minds of Bob and the girls, but then my own thoughts would always pull me back to praying for Taylor's life. Just as the tide comes in and out, washing away the sand, I needed to wash away any negative thoughts and just enjoy the moment, like Taylor could do. It was difficult for me, but for her, it seemed easy.

The next day we decided to explore the island by helicopter. As we waited in line, Ryan was visibly nervous; she wasn't a fan of heights and often got motion sickness. The sight of the prior passengers somewhat reassured us as they jumped off the helicopter, huge smiles on of their faces. Wind gusts circulating from the propellers sent our hair flying and our hearts racing, and nearly knocked Corey over. With hand gestures, Bob signaled to all his girls, including me, to remain calm. Of course, Taylor jumped in the front seat with the pilot as the four of us gathered in the back.

The pilot dipped down and around, showing us the many and varied vistas of Kona, an island stitched together like a beautiful quilt. In stark comparison to the lava fields and arid plains we had seen at the airport, we took in the breathtaking coastline, an array of magnificent blues and greens, huge volcanoes spitting out small amounts of hot molten lava, and a multitude of waterfalls nestled throughout lush valleys. This was Mother Nature at her best, a perfect, living landscape.

Suddenly, Taylor grabbed the vomit bag, an abrupt reminder of cancer amidst all the natural beauty surrounding us. My heart raced. But this time it was just motion sickness. *Nothing to worry about; get your mind back in the moment,* I commanded myself.

Later in the day, we explored the beach, but we were not allowed to swim in the ocean due to the enormous strength of the tide. Gigantic turtles lay in the bright sunshine, seemingly asleep. "Tales and Cor, don't touch the turtles," I warned, but they couldn't resist poking sticks at them, ignoring my pleas. One of the turtles began creeping along the sand so slowly it seemed it could barely hold the weight of its gigantic shell. As I watched him amble along, I was reminded that we share our world and all of its burdens with so many of God's creatures. Like the turtle, I carried a gigantic weight on my back, a burden only God could explain. I prayed that one day it would all make sense.

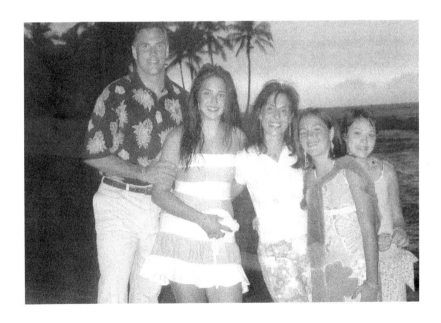

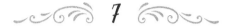

Battle Mode

*When you have exhausted all possibilities,
remember this–you haven't.*

–Thomas Edison

Forget It, I'm Wearing Sweatpants!

By May 2006, Taylor looked like the picture of health. Her olive skin tone was restored; her eyes were gleaming; her hair had grown in; her body was beginning to fill out; and the suffering in her eyes had dissipated. She looked radiant and was preparing for a return to competitive sports in the fall. This summer would be her first real summer in three years, and she was full of plans; she had already selected a teen tour of the West Coast.

Taylor had also just passed her two-year remission date. We could hardly believe how blessed we were. On a notepad, I happily scribbled down names in anticipation of giving her a big surprise party. That idea was quickly shot down when I spoke to her friends, all of whom reminded me, "Tales will be mortified."

I was so ecstatic with the news I forgot that Taylor would hate the attention. Silently, I applauded her victory.

According to schedule, Taylor was due for scans. It was a huge milestone for her to pass her one-year remission date, let alone her two-year, and we had become used to good news. As usual, fear was still lurking, but Bob reassured me, "Don't worry; if the cancer was going to come back, it would've already." I was content with that reasoning.

The following week, Taylor's scans showed activity in her left adrenal gland, almost certainly a recurrence. That site had been suspicious at the time of her first diagnosis but had remained dormant or dead since our early success at Columbia. We feared Tales was about to start reliving the nightmare.

We immediately went into cancer mode, trying to schedule surgery that week. Taylor's favorite surgeon at Columbia, Dr. Rubin, was on vacation and wouldn't return until Friday. Taylor flat out refused to have surgery on Friday because it was International Day at school, and she insisted, "I'm not missing Friday night out with my friends." She wanted a surgeon who could operate on Thursday. We scheduled surgery accordingly.

Dr. Rubin, still on vacation, called me at home, angry as a hornet. "You can't wait a day?" I instantly responded, "No, Taylor has a life!" From that day forward, he never spoke to us again. I was shocked that an adult dealing with a kid with cancer was behaving like a petulant child, letting his ego get in the way. Likewise, Taylor was terribly upset and truly baffled. She was used to having excellent relationships with her doctors and couldn't get her mind around this one.

The surgery removed one of Taylor's adrenal glands; luckily, we have two adrenal glands, and people can live perfectly normal lives with just one. Tales qualified for "minimally invasive surgery," or laparoscopic surgery, which accomplishes surgery through tubes inserted at several spots in the abdomen. This approach shortens the time of recovery and lowers the risk of complication and infection in most people. However, we were cautioned that although the incision was minimal, the tissue trauma and damage to internal organs would be the same, and it was no minor event. For most people, it probably would have been a pretty big deal, and certainly we didn't take it lightly, but on the Taylor scale, it was about a five or six. She spent one night in the hospital, the night of our twenty-first wedding anniversary, after a successful removal of the tumor, with no evidence of spread outside the local area.

The pain made it impossible for Tales to go to school the next morning, but she managed to get discharged that afternoon in time to go out Friday night. With continuing incision pain and a huge belly from the air inserted in her stomach during laparoscopic surgery, this would be no easy feat. With trepidation, I walked into her room to find jeans all over the floor. Flustered, she screamed, "I can't fit into any of them because of my huge stomach!" Tears welled as she turned to me and said, "Forget it; I'm wearing sweatpants," and immediately got on her cell phone to make plans. I stood inside her bedroom door and stared out the window, thinking, *How can she possibly endure more surgery and more suffering and still go on without acknowledging it?* As it turned out, she had a wonderful time that night. Fun was a magnet for Tales.

The biopsy came back positive. Cancer had bulldozed its way back into our lives. Bob and I sunk deeply into our chairs, our eyes misty and glazed over. Reality had not yet fully hit. Taylor was outside with her friends in the hot tub. We felt she should know right away. Were we insane to interrupt her time with her friends? Maybe we were the ones who needed her support and courage. When we called her inside to tell her the news, she looked at us blankly, said, "Okay," and left.

An avalanche of hot tears streamed down my face as we watched her jump right back in with her friends as if nothing had happened. We wondered, *How does she compartmentalize like that?* Cancer, like a hurricane with one-hundred-mile winds, was about to wreak havoc and knock us down again, and we knew it. We kept telling ourselves we were lucky because she relapsed to a single site, a tumor on her adrenal gland, when many times cancer comes raging back more aggressively. We were determined to look at the glass as half full.

When Tales was first diagnosed, we knew very little about her disease, the ordeals to follow, the treatments she would endure, and what surgery really meant. By now we knew exactly what was coming, and the prospect of entering the war zone and doing battle again felt inconceivable. True to form, the first person to snap back into battle mode and resign herself to round two of this title fight was Taylor. Taylor just looked her disease in the eye and kept fighting.

She was a force of nature. We couldn't comprehend how she could look past the hurdles and concentrate on the next item on her life's agenda while being subjected to so much suffering—and to do it while giving you a good slap in the face, occasionally.

We soon realized that no matter what we did, so much was out of our hands. But that helplessness lit a fire in me, a fire that burned so deeply it brought me right into the next day's war zone. It gave me the ability to never give up and the strength to endure.

We waited several days longer to receive the pathology report than we ever had before. The doctors asked for slides from Taylor's original pathology at Sloan and brought in several other doctors before coming to a conclusion. The appearance of Taylor's cancer cells seemed to be very different from the classic appearance of osteosarcoma, which is what Sloan diagnosed her with three years prior. Instead, the cells resembled chondrosarcoma (a cousin of osteosarcoma that arises from cartilage) and were "mesenchymal" in type, meaning they arose from a primitive type of cell stemming from connective tissue. Nevertheless, the consensus was that this was not a new cancer, but a recurrence of the original cancer.

Once again, Bob searched desperately for a cutting-edge protocol, preferably one that would attack chemical and biological pathways. He got many opinions—all informed guesses.

Taylor had no intention of canceling her planned West Coast teen tour with her friends. That meant starting chemotherapy during school finals. She took an exam in the morning and came leaping back into the car, excited just like the other kids to be done—except instead of going out to lunch with her friends, she was going to the hospital for more chemo. Her teachers and friends were not aware that Taylor was on chemotherapy or that she had relapsed. She had made a firm decision not to tell anyone this time, and no one had to know; this chemotherapy was not supposed to result in hair loss. She was determined to be normal.

It also meant we had to find a way for her to secretly continue chemotherapy during her teen tour. We planned our schedule: each week, I would fly out and stay in a hotel close by, so no one would know I was there. I would take her off the program for a few days, bring her to the hospital for chemo, stay with her until the side effects wore off, and return her to the program. I'd then return home myself.

The day before she left, her doctors decided to add a new drug to her regiment, one I was told to administer with rubber gloves. Starting a new drug, with potentially severe side effects, on the day before she was leaving was more than Taylor could handle. The only reason her doctors allowed it was that Taylor was Taylor. But this time she became frightened. Nine hours before her plane was to depart, she came to me crying, "Mommy, can I stay home?"

Corey was at sleep-away camp, so Ryan was supposed to be the only one home during the weeks Taylor was away. She was finally going to get time alone with us, to actually be our priority and not be the less-important one, the one who couldn't complain or be upset or be ungrateful because things were so much worse for Taylor. When she heard Taylor wasn't going on her trip, she didn't say much, but I could tell it was a crushing disappointment, like her summer had been canceled.

I felt so bad for Ryan. I called my friend Janet, bawling about our change in circumstances. She immediately said, "Can Ryan join us on our trip?" Janet was leaving that same day for Italy on a celebratory fiftieth-birthday family vacation. A barrage of tears cascaded down my cheeks as I thought about what a generous, kind, and loving person Janet was to all of us. She was truly a second sister.

We couldn't get a ticket on the same flight as Janet's, and there was no time to get Ryan an international cell phone. So we arranged for Ryan, who was barely seventeen at the time, to wait in the Rome airport for Janet, as Janet's flight was landing a bit later. From start to finish, everything happened in less than three hours. By then, we had all developed the idea that everything in our lives was insanity, so in a way, nothing was.

Today, I would never be able to book a flight, pack and drive to the airport with three hours' notice, and send a teenager on a plane unescorted to a foreign country. But back then, we were in cancer mode; anything was possible, and we wouldn't let anything stop us from embracing any and all opportunities for sunshine amidst the gloom. We set out to find the lemonade in lemons, our motto throughout, which may have been the most important aspect of Taylor's treatment plan.

While Ryan was in Italy, I spontaneously scheduled a four-day trip to the Caribbean island of Anguilla, between treatments, with Taylor's friend Jenny, whom she had known since third grade and whose boundless energy shone as brightly as her sun-kissed blonde hair. The trip allowed us to forget our medical challenges and instead focus on making the perfect sandcastle.

Taylor, Jenny, and I arrived, checked in, and headed for the beach. Like typical teenagers, the girls immediately began scoping out cute guys. There were none at the present moment, but they saw some kids out on a huge float that was a bit of a distance away. We all dove in and swam out. Taylor struggled, but she made it, and although it proved fruitless in the cute guy department, we laughed together, and Tales felt a tremendous sense of accomplishment.

On our way back to New York, while going through customs, Jenny decided to push the customs agent's buttons to see how far she could get. She placed her foot right over the line that says, "Do not put your foot over this line until you are called," and then took a picture of her foot crossing the line, even though cameras are forbidden in customs. When Jen got caught, it was hard for me to keep a straight face, but I knew I had no choice. I quickly deleted the picture in front of the agent.

In the customs exit line, tired and slaphappy, all three of us put on our sunglasses, as a goof. The agent very seriously asked us to all remove our glasses and asked, "What's your reason for traveling?" We replied, "Just to have fun." He wasn't too pleased with that answer, so I quickly moved both of them along. Knowing she would soon be in agony from chemo the next day, it brought me great joy to see Taylor enjoying the silly things in life, and I couldn't help but join in. I, too, lost my sense of being the adult and joined in with the kids. Everyone needs moments of sheer happiness, blue skies, and rainbows.

Pizza "Party"

As August 2006 was winding down, we found ourselves in our favorite room in our home, which had now become the room with all the computers. We used to call it the playroom, as it had once been filled with brightly colored toys of every shape and size. It was now beautifully decorated in hues of beige and green and housed two large credenzas with desktop computers, a desk for laptops, a pullout couch, and a television.

Taylor was not feeling well, complaining about pain surrounding her belly button, and Ryan was writing her college essays. I felt like a jumping bean, as one moment Ryan asked me to read her essays and the next Taylor begged me to come sit with her on the couch. My chair rolled back and forth between the two girls while my eyes rolled back in my head. They were in such different places, yet they both begged for my attention.

Eventually, Taylor won out, which left Ryan, once again, on her own. Ryan was rightfully upset. It was totally unfair. Writing college essays is one of the most demanding and dreaded tasks a high school student endures. My very being was split in two, but I had no choice but to tend to Tales. As always, Bob came to Ryan's rescue.

Taylor's pain worsened as the night rolled on. We couldn't identify the cause or see anything on her skin. But, remember, this is the kid who rarely complained—and the mother who constantly worried. I called the hospital, and the on-call doctor nonchalantly said, "Bring her into clinic tomorrow." Because Tales had no visible indications of illness, they said to watch her and see what happens. I snapped, "Really? Just let her suffer?" The medical world had once again served us the "cold freeze." Taylor slept in my arms that night, just as any baby would, cuddling with her mommy but writhing in pain.

In the morning, her skin was slightly red around her belly button. We flew to clinic. The doctors thought she might have a cellulitis infection. Cellulitis is an acute infection of resistant bacteria that can enter through breaks in the skin and is a common result of surgery. Although it can be worrisome, her doctors concluded that the infection was minor, as the redness was barely noticeable. Taylor received a dose of IV antibiotics and pain meds and was sent home.

I was skeptical, as Taylor's pain had reached a high level, but she reassured me, "Mommy, trust the doctors; I will be okay." As the day progressed into the evening, the pain worsened and a bright-red oval appeared around her belly button, where the scab from her adrenal surgery was still evident. By evening, Tales could barely walk. An emergency room visit was warranted, no matter what the doctors said. I called the hospital and calmly stated, "We are en route to the hospital. Expect Taylor Matthews," and hung up before they could say a word.

The doctors soon figured out that the cellulitis was a side effect of her laparoscopic surgery performed through her navel three months earlier. The incision in her belly button had never properly healed, due to her low immune system. They admitted Taylor to the hospital and put her on heavy doses of antibiotics. As the days rolled on, it got worse. Each day, the doctors drew a pen line on Taylor's belly to mark the size of the infection. It grew, day after day. Clearly, the antibiotics were not working.

Every morning, the doctors rounded, looked at her chart, conferred silently, and changed her IV antibiotics to ones I knew were getting stronger and stronger. They barely said a word and refused to make the slightest eye contact. Thanks to heavy doses of pain medications, Taylor was in high spirits, and I was determined to spend every minute having fun with her, adopting her attitude of making the most out of life, putting aside the bad, and only focusing on the positive. But I knew the situation was dire and urgent.

I feared Taylor could die. Doctors from the surgical team, the infectious disease team, the oncology team, and the attendants on the floor were all visiting, but they couldn't find an antibiotic that worked. Not one of them was honest with us. But the fight was never over in our minds. Bob refused to accept what we thought the doctors were not humane enough to tell us.

When I demanded to speak with the doctors to get a straight answer, the nurses treated me like I was insane, inappropriate, and annoying. Their voices droned, "This is a hospital with a lot of patients. The doctors are busy; they have already seen Taylor, and they will get back to you when they can." I was screaming at deaf ears, and with a rush of adrenaline, I hollered, "Please page the doctors now! We need help!" But they refused to do any more than they had already done.

The next morning, as usual, her doctors said nothing and hastily exited as quickly as they came in. I told Taylor I would be right back and sprinted to catch the team of doctors before they saw the next patient. Standing tall, with anger and fear emanating from every pore, I demanded, "Excuse me. May I speak with you a moment?" They turned to me with blank stares and then instinctively averted their eyes. I knew I would only have their attention for a minute, so my questions came out in rapid fire: "What is my daughter's actual prognosis? I know the antibiotics are not working. What does that mean? What is our next step? Why is the infection spreading? Have you given her the most broad-spectrum antibiotics you have? Are they the strongest ones you have?" And then I shouted my final question: "Is my daughter dying? Please, please tell me the truth."

I wasn't prepared for their answer. One doctor replied, "Yes, Mrs. Matthews, if the infection continues, your daughter will die from it." The air escaped my lungs as I bent over, dry heaving in the middle of the hallway.

Desperate for a solution, I reached out to Christine, part PhD, part coach, part child psychologist, friend to dozens of kids at Columbia, and our favorite alternative medicine therapist. She assured me she had an herbal treatment—"a rain bath," as she called it—to clear bacterial infections. She arrived, towels in hand, with a huge box of herbal liquids, and went to work, rubbing Taylor with herbs and then covering her with a combination of hot and cold towels. The aroma of a fresh pizza filled our room. As Christine carried out her routine, she and Taylor carried on their usual banter, which always included a lot of laughter.

At this point I feared death could be imminent. Again, I felt as though I was standing out of my body behind a glass wall, watching Taylor and Christine scene-by-scene, as the movie reel played before my eyes. How would it end? I could see them laughing and noticed Taylor's muscles relaxing from the massage and warmth of the hot towels. Christine glanced at me from time to time, her eyes reflecting the gravity of the situation. At the same time, her expressions were comforting and indicated to me that she believed all could be well. I have no idea how long Christine stayed with us, but I do remember it was a Friday night, and as always, she was not leaving until she felt she had done everything humanly possible. Through her years of dedication and service, Christine sacrificed everything in her life to help children with cancer.

The next morning, Taylor awoke without pain. Knowing her life was hanging in the wind, I lifted her shirt and glanced at her belly with all the courage I could muster, praying and hoping the infection had not grown larger. I couldn't believe my eyes. The infection, as indicated by the size of the redness around her belly button, had shrunk from the size of softball to the size of a dime. I was speechless, with my heart in my mouth. Taylor was going to live! As fast as my feet could take me, I ran to get the nurses. The doctors followed quickly behind. All were thrilled but refused to acknowledge that Christine's "rain bath" had anything to do with it.

I didn't care what they thought; all that mattered was Taylor was well! Taylor had no idea how close she had come to death. Every time I smell pizza, its aroma brings me right back to my memories of Taylor's rain bath and how it saved her life. I will never underestimate the importance of using alternative therapies. Or the importance of people dedicated to kids, like Christine.

Another Hurdle

In September 2006, Ryan was starting her senior year of high school. She had already been accepted to Wake Forest University through early admission and was thrilled to be leaving the stress of the college process behind and going to her first choice. Corey was starting her first year of junior high as a seventh grader and joining both of her sisters at the same school for the first time. Tales was getting her wish to be a "normal" kid, laying out her back-to-school clothes and joining her friends for classes, lunch, and, most important, constant chatter about the boys.

Also around this time, Tales was due to receive her normal ninety-day scans. We had built some confidence that, even though cancer had appeared in her adrenal gland, the most dangerous "dead" tumors still in her lungs were under control. We had had the option to remove these dead tumors when Taylor went into remission, but we declined, as she had already lost too much of her lung capacity.

To our shock, the scan results showed that one of the larger nodules in Taylor's lungs had grown. Apparently, that so-called dead tumor was very much alive, and this made us wonder if some of Taylor's tumors had always been only dormant, rather than dead. Bob had learned how to read scans and was now reading them every time they were run. Bob saw some additional suspicious areas beyond the one enlarged nodule the radiologist saw in the scan. He pushed the doctors to explain, but they insisted that nothing appeared strange.

Taylor had relapsed for a second time in four months, and this time only six weeks after chemo. Bob redoubled his efforts, speaking with doctors from all around the country, to keep our approach creative, aggressive, and founded on the best thinking anywhere in the world. He was back to working at his day job and researching throughout the night.

In that research, he came across several articles written by a leading name in the field of pediatric cancer, Dr. Peter Anderson, whose work at the Mayo Clinic had helped to shape our decisions back in 2003. Dr. Anderson was now at MD Anderson in Houston, one of the most well-regarded cancer hospitals in the world and a leading research facility. Within three days, we were on a plane to Houston.

MD Anderson is like no other hospital we have ever visited. It is run with the efficiency of a Swiss bank. Our itinerary at the hospital for the coming days listed every test and appointment scheduled, its location, and the telephone number to call with any questions.

Upon arrival, our senses were heightened by the masterful sound of the piano echoing throughout the lobby. For a moment, I felt like a little girl again, hearing my grandfather's fingers dance up and down the ivory keys that had resided in our living room.

We spent two days with Dr. Anderson, days that were both remarkable and sobering. After running through a litany of tests that checked and rechecked the scans done at Columbia, he sat down to review and explain the scans by showing us the actual films—quite a stark change from other hospitals where we got minimal information from the radiology reports. While we were waiting, a medical resident shadowing Dr. Anderson did a cursory exam on Tales. He stopped during the exam and asked Dr. Anderson to feel the left side of Taylor's neck where her lymph nodes were located. There was a palpable hard lump under the surface of the skin. You didn't need to be an oncologist to know this was a very bad sign.

I have to admit that our guard was down when we arrived in Houston. After all, we had just had a scan a week before at Columbia. How much bad news could there be? As it turned out, plenty. When we sat to review the results, Dr. Anderson pointed out a bright spot, just where Bob had seen one on the

Columbia scan. Taylor had a tumor growing on her right adrenal that had clearly grown right through treatment. We didn't know whether to cry or scream.

The news got worse. Dr. Anderson pointed out several other growing tumors. We were speechless. We couldn't fathom why the Columbia radiologist hadn't articulated any of this a week earlier. We learned the hard way the importance of investigating the doctor you are working with, regardless of the hospital you are being treated at. We suspect they saw what Bob saw but focused us on only what they wanted to address.

In short order, we decided to get all future scans at MD Anderson. We also found Dr. Anderson's thinking to be creative, aggressive, and refreshing. He spoke the plain, unvarnished truth but had great enthusiasm for next steps to help Tales. He had more ideas than we could actually execute at one time!

Due to the sad state of oncology, all doctors and all hospitals don't have the same information. We asked him to consult on the case permanently. Part of the blunt assessment we received from him came in the form of a comment and a question. He said he was troubled by the behavior of the tumors, and he asked us repeatedly whether we were sure that Taylor had osteosarcoma. No one had ever outright challenged the diagnosis, despite the significant delay and debate over pathology after Taylor's adrenal surgery. However, upon hearing that Sloan had made the diagnosis, he dropped the discussion, commenting, "They certainly should know osteosarcoma when they see it."

At this point, opinions diverged on what to do next. We clearly needed to add and change treatments, and we needed a plan to eliminate the newly reactivated tumors. Dr. Anderson wanted to charge ahead with treatment and discuss surgical solutions. Dr. Garvin was anxious to get a biopsy of the tumors in Taylor's chest but was less interested in surgery. Dr. La Quaglia from Sloan was interested in a sample, either through biopsy or actual surgery. Ultimately, Dr. La Quaglia arranged for a biopsy; it was now three-and-a-half years after Taylor's original diagnosis. We were blessed that our doctors were willing to collaborate.

One afternoon at Columbia, I passed Dr. Garvin in the hallway on my way to the vending machine, and he said three words I'll never forget: "Taylor was misdiagnosed." My breath stopped short, and I screamed, "What?" He didn't reply but instead handed me a black and white pathology report from Sloan:

"Previous material was reviewed, and in retrospect, the appearance is consistent with mesenchymal chondrosarcoma, rather than small cell osteosarcoma."

Tears were flowing uncontrollably; my stomach was calling for a toilet, or at least a garbage can, in which to vomit. I was barely capable of walking. Human error again? Hadn't all the proper and necessary steps to diagnose her type of cancer been taken? Where were all the checks and balances? Over and over, Taylor's life had lain in the hands of one individual—in this case, a pathologist. Given that Taylor was diagnosed at Memorial Sloan Kettering, we never second-guessed it. Clearly, like most, we had relied on their reputation, but even the best hospitals can employ people who make mistakes. If you are facing cancer or any malady, challenge everything and everyone.

I returned with a handful of goodies, but Taylor could tell something was wrong. I had been crying and was visibly shaken. There was nothing left to do but tell her the news. "Taylor, sweetheart, I am so sorry. Dr. Garvin just told me you don't have osteosarcoma." I was mad and ready to sue the hospital, the doctors—everybody! "You have a cancer called mesenchymal chondrosarcoma."

I cannot recall her expression, but her response echoes in my heart to this day. She said calmly, "Okay, it's water under the bridge. Where do we go from here?" Then, in an extremely stern voice, like she was the parent and I was the child, she added, "Mommy, I can see you are enraged. Never sue Sloan. That would only be negative energy. I need you to stay positive so I can get better." We fell into each other's arms, and for once, she let me cry. My heart was bleeding, but the pure love we shared at that moment will carry me through for the rest of my life.

Another Happy Birthday

After a grand fifteenth birthday celebration at the Gansevoort hotel in the meatpacking district of New York City, with eight of Taylor's closest friends, it was time once again for chemo. Unfortunately, she needed chemo on her actual birthday. Taylor and I had fought hard with her doctors to reschedule, but this time it was impossible. When the day came, she was so beaten up by side effects that she easily relented. Our birthday family tradition was a breakfast of Dunkin Donuts with candles in them. She couldn't hide her discomfort. She looked up at me with listless brown eyes, smiled, looked at the candles as long as she could, and then ran to the bathroom to vomit. Taylor never rallied that day.

I didn't concentrate on how ill she was on her fifteenth birthday, but rather on how much fun she had had at her party a few days prior. She and her girlfriends were all piled up on one bed in the hotel, giggling and chatting like typical teenagers. That was when she told them, without missing a beat, that she had relapsed. They were stunned, but Taylor wouldn't allow it to put a damper on her night. Her *joie de vivre* was so contagious that, despite the news, everyone forgot their woes and continued to party into the night.

I Love Your Hair!

Taylor pleaded, "Nothing is going to get in the way, Susssan, of us going to London for Thanksgiving!" Andrea and her family had been living there for the past year. Obliging Tales this time was going to be more complicated than it might sound, even for us. The week of Thanksgiving, Taylor was due for a five-day chemo cycle, which needed to be administered in a clinical setting, so we would have to find a hospital in London. Not only that, but we were also scheduled to visit MD Anderson in Houston that week. "Piece of cake," she said. I thought, *Really, Tales? It's a piece of cake to have treatment in three hospitals in three cities on two continents in one week?* But I knew my girl, and this was definitely in her wheelhouse.

Taylor arrived in London with some seriously screwed-up chemo hair, all chopped and frizzy. Wide-eyed, the first words out of Samantha were, "Taylor! I *love* your hair." She was absolutely serious. It gave us all a laugh and the relief we needed. The next morning, Samantha roped Taylor into waking up early and going to her international nursery school to explain Thanksgiving to the foreign children. Taylor was overjoyed.

After chemo at London's Great Ormond Street Hospital, where we were treated like royalty, Taylor frolicked down the streets of London, hand in hand with Samantha, without a care in the world. Later that day, as part of "The Wild Cats" club invented by Tales and Corey, Taylor taught her little cousin the art of a perfect prank. Together, they took the cookies that Andrea had bought for everyone and replaced all the icing with toothpaste.

Thanksgiving had always involved pranks. Years earlier, when the kids were small, our extended family had gathered in the dining room, as usual, to voice our gratitude. In unison, giggling, my girls chanted, "We are thankful that Mommy made us *penne alla vodka* so we don't have to eat turkey." Then the girls surreptitiously climbed under the dining room table and tied all the males' shoelaces together. Without being seen, they got right back in their chairs and joined in the festivities, until my dad got up from the table.

At first, he couldn't figure out why he couldn't move his feet and stumbled a bit. We looked at him, thinking maybe he had had too much wine. "Christ, my shoelaces are tied together," grumbled Dad. Now we really thought he must be drunk—that is, until we all looked at his shoes (and by "we" I mean everyone, including my girls, who expressed serious looks of concern). Before my brother got up, he looked down at his shoelaces, and sure enough, they were also tied together. I'm not sure what the others were thinking, but personally I laughed until the tears started rolling.

The London Thanksgiving weekend ended way too quickly. Time always flew at an alarming rate when our family was with Andrea's. The girls were so sad to part ways, but tears turned to sass when Samantha, hands on hips, admonished, "Aunt Sue! You always make my mommy cry when you say goodbye to each other." We all embraced and then hopped in a black taxi heading for Heathrow Airport, with heads down, tear-stained cheeks, and hearts full of memories, laughter, and love. I know that love was very much a part of what healed Taylor during her journey.

Christmas by the Sea

In December 2006, the girls were seventeen, fifteen, and twelve. We spent a magnificent Christmas at The Cloisters in Sea Island, Georgia, a place we had come to call home. Bob and I had visited Sea Island in the 1980s, pre-children. On our first day, while walking out of our room, we nearly bumped into a member of the housekeeping staff and were instantly mesmerized. "Good morning, ma'am and sir," she drawled. "Is there anything we can do for you?" The southern charm of Sea Island was foreign to us, me being a native New Yorker and Bob being from the outskirts of Philadelphia. Bob whispered to me, "Do you think they want something from us?" I shrugged. That was the beginning of the Matthews family tradition of vacationing at Sea Island.

When we arrived, the same friendly, gentlemanly, burly southern bellmen, who had worked at Sea Island for over thirty years, greeted us by name and extended a huge welcome. Although we had vacationed at Sea Island dozens of times throughout the years, it was our first Christmas there, just the five of us. As we entered the main building, we were stunned by the beauty and elegance that lay before us. I glanced around the enormous lobby, and the smell of freshly cut pine enveloped me as my eyes soaked in the exquisite beauty of the live decorations. Numerous imposing but dazzling Christmas trees stood throughout, almost as tall as the three-story lobby. A festoon of lavish green vines adorned the grand staircase, and an abundance of floral arrangements displayed on every table created the aura of a fairytale.

We ventured up to our suite and were greeted by soft white lights shining from a small but perfectly shaped Christmas tree that had been placed in our room. Alongside the tree lay a large straw basket filled with finely crafted, colorful ornaments representing themes of the Cloister. The girls beamed and then quickly grimaced, realizing that colorful ornaments, no matter how cute, would never make it onto my tree. We all started laughing together, without having to say a word. They knew that I had shipped to the hotel dozens of bleached sand dollars, which would later be attached to the tree, ever so meticulously, with beautiful ruby-red ribbons. We had found most of those sand dollars in years past at Sea Island.

During many of our summer trips to Sea Island, the girls took a jeep train ride along the seemingly always-sunny beach to discover the vegetation and beds of sea life. Naturally, the hotel had timed the ride perfectly so that the tide would be low when the kids got out of the jeep, making the sand dollars buried in the deeper area of the ocean ripe for the picking. These living creatures hold rich symbolism and hidden gems. The legend of the sand dollar tells us that on one side, the Easter lily with a star in its center represents the star of Bethlehem, and on the other is a poinsettia, the traditional Christmas flower. And when you break open a sand dollar, to our perpetual amazement, five tiny and perfectly shaped dove shells emerge. According to the legend, the doves spread good will and peace.

The day after Christmas, we headed back to the airport to pick up Corey and Taylor's friends, Julie and Jenny. The week went by without drama, rather odd for teenagers. One evening I walked into the girls' room to find Corey and Julie bouncing on the beds, with wet towels, clothes, and empty water bottles scattered on every inch of the floor. I thought to myself, *Oh, boy, they are having fun, but this is not okay.* Just as I was about to admonish them, I caught sight of Taylor and Jenny, hovering in the corner, speaking in hushed tones. I could see that whatever they were talking about was important, but their huge grins also told me they were up to no good.

I walked over and said, "What's up?" Instantly, both girls became silent, diverting their eyes away from me. I said, "Come on, you can tell me anything." They immediately burst into uproarious laughter. Jenny gushed out, "Taylor likes this kid Jordan and is hoping to make out with him on New Year's. She already hooked up with him, but he was too drunk to remember." I replied, "Really, Tales, isn't it your tradition to kiss Allen every New Year's?" referring to another teenage boy in our neighborhood. Taylor replied sarcastically, "Oh, Mommy, of course I'll keep my promise to Allen, but I also want to kiss Jordan." I replied nonchalantly, "Good luck with that, Tales," not knowing how much she really cared for this new boy. She was living a normal teenage life, full of gossip, boys, and drama.

"Who is Jordan?" I asked. Taylor blurted out, "You remember the family, Mommy! Corey used to be friends with his little sister Olivia." I thought back many years and quickly put together the pieces. I remembered Jordan as a cutie pie, whose ocean-blue eyes, even at six years old, revealed his mischievous personality. Little did I know how on point my assessment was!

The Wizard

Not long after that fateful exchange, Taylor came home one day and announced that Jordan was her boyfriend.

Ever since Tales was a little tot, she had always wanted a boyfriend. My dad, whom she called "Pop-Pop," used to tease her about her pretend boyfriend "Barnett." Every time he saw her, his first question was, "Taylor, how is Barnett?" to which she would respond, in her tiny voice, "BAW-nett" and I did this, and we did that, describing tall tales about their adventures. Taylor's imagination was vivid, and she was always up for sharing her stories.

One time Taylor brought Andrea up to her room and, with tremendous mischief in her grin, asked her to sit on the bed. In hushed tones and with the cutest New York accent, she leaned in and said, "Aunt Annie! I tell everyone Baw-nett is not my boy-fwend." She paused for dramatic emphasis and then shouted, "*But he really is!*" Aunt Andrea had no idea that Barnett was a figment of Taylor and Pop-Pop's imagination until a decade later.

At first, Tales wasn't sure if Jordan knew about her past or current battle with cancer. I thought, *In the small town that we live in, how could he not know?* I imagine she was somewhat in denial, simply craving some normalcy. Nothing about having cancer at fifteen and entering into a relationship was normal. Taylor delicately explained the situation to him. Telling people she had cancer was always, understandably, very difficult.

The Jordan tale has many twists and turns, but I have to admit that he accepted and participated in Taylor's pain, Taylor's treatment, and Taylor's life in a way that is truly commendable and heartwarming for anyone, let alone a teenage boy. Remarkably, he saw her for the person she was, not for the disease she had. Likewise, she adored him, despite his own difficulties, and her belief in him truly catapulted him to a new level. He learned to believe in himself. The two of them were like Felix and Oscar, a very unlikely couple, but eventually they became inseparable.

At fifteen, Jordan was a cute kid, on the shorter side, with a sandy-brown buzz cut and a personality hotter than a jalapeno pepper. He was also famously known, at least in our house, for his horrendous clothes. Every day he wore the same-looking pair of baggy jeans. He had an orange-and-grey-striped sweatshirt and old-man poncho that Taylor hated and threw out many times in his garbage, only to have him fetch them back out.

He was not known for his academic accomplishments or his motivation to achieve good grades. I believe life was too much fun for him to care about school, and he had legitimate learning challenges he had been working on for years. Taylor, on the other hand, was extremely academic, despite her lack of attendance in school. She influenced Jordan in many ways, but none more than his schoolwork. Years later our superintendent confirmed, "We all believe that Taylor turned Jordan around academically."

Jordan would arrive at our house at the end of every school day at exactly a quarter past three. I enjoyed joking around with him and always offered him an after-school snack, but before he could accept it, we would hear Taylor screaming from her room, "Susssan! Let him go." Jordan would smile and dart up the stairs as quickly as possible.

Most days when I would wander into Taylor's room, he would be sitting at her desk with his back to her, doing his homework. She would sport a huge grin while lying on her bed making faces behind his back and mouthing to me, "Can you believe it?" She was not going to have a slacker for a boyfriend, and she was determined to change the teachers' opinions of him.

Coming to our house after school did not sit well with Jordan's mother, Robbin. He was a junior in high school, getting ready for college applications. Knowing his previous antics and varied excuses about avoiding homework, I imagine she didn't believe he was doing homework. She suggested that they needed to break up. Taylor took her to task big time. She belted out, "Mommy, can you believe Robbin has the nerve to suggest we break up? Who is she kidding?" As she ranted, words kept spilling off her tongue as she forcefully clicked open her laptop and aggressively typed an email to Robbin. "Mommy, I know I should be respectful of Jordan's mom, but she cannot do this to us!" I have to admit, I was hysterically laughing inside as I read the email and unsuccessfully tried to get her to soften the tone.

Together, Jordan and Taylor wrote the words for his senior year high school yearbook that would appear next to his picture: "Their once was a boy, this boy needed help. Just then a magical wizard appeared. The wiz said he would help him but he had to show him other people who would help him. [Jordan speaks about many people.] Next the wiz took him to this Gr8 girl, Taylor Matthews, whom the boy took to be his princess. He thnx TM and her family. Then the boy got up from his excellent adventure and looked in the mirror and realized he had turned into the wiz because of all these people he had turned into a better person. Good luck to everyone and I hope that if anyone is ever in trouble they find themselves a wizard."

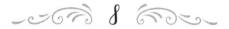

Living Out of Bounds

You gain strength, courage, and confidence in every experience by which you really stop to face fear in the face. You are able to say to yourself, "I lived through the horror. I can take the next thing that comes along."

–Eleanor Roosevelt

When the Red Wristband Didn't Sound the Bells

Three weeks into her relationship with Jordan, Taylor was scheduled for a very complicated surgery at Weill Cornell that would begin with a thoracotomy and end with surgery to excise an infection along her scoliosis rods. The night before surgery, Taylor's room was filled with friends. From down the hall, I could hear chatting and boisterous laughter. Taylor's friends had decided to have an autograph party, but instead of autographing a get-well pillow or a T-shirt, they autographed Taylor herself. When I entered her room, she rolled up her pajamas, laughing hysterically, and exclaimed, "Look at me!" She was covered in pen with stories of love and well wishes resembling those on the back pages of a signed yearbook.

Prior to surgery, Taylor's surgeon rolled his eyes, exclaiming, "My nurses have FedEx boxes going all over the country with specific instructions. How many places in the world are you sending samples of Taylor's tumor?" I snarled and spit out, "We are sending it to many places. Are we overworking your nurses, or trying to save Taylor's life?" Tumors can be analyzed many different ways at different institutions to identify biological markers and target treatments that may be more successful. The more opinions you have, the better the chances are of having the best treatment for your child's cancer. But our plan was mostly about saving tumor samples for treatments not available in the United States.

Bob came out of the OR after Taylor was peacefully under general anesthesia, and we made our way to the ever-familiar waiting room, where all we could do was wait, cry, and pray; pray, cry, and wait. The surgery was estimated to take approximately six hours. You could imagine our surprise when, after about only four hours, Taylor's orthopedic surgeon Dr. David walked in.

Dr. David, a tall teddy-bear-of-a-man with graying temples and a huge presence, was supposed to do the scoliosis part of Taylor's surgery. He looked too fresh to have just completed a scoliosis repair. Instinctively, my heart beat so furiously I felt I could almost see it thumping through my shirt. He was looking down at the floor, so that all we could see were the deep lines creasing his forehead. Gravely he explained, "Taylor had an allergic reaction to an antibiotic she received during surgery, and we had to abort."

Apparently, when Dr. David entered the OR after the thoracic portion of her surgery was completed, he noticed Taylor was developing a rash and her breathing had become short. He immediately recognized anaphylactic shock, a possibly life-threatening reaction to an allergen that can come on very quickly. This was about as scary a development as one could conjure.

The looks on our faces were probably twisted, contorted, and sickening, like morphing monsters in a horror show. My lips were trembling, eyes welling with tears, and I felt paralyzed with fear. I couldn't speak a word. Bob took hold of the situation. "Is she okay?" was all he could muster and the only question that mattered. Dr. David responded yes. That was all I needed to hear, and my fear turned into red, hot anger, boiling over out of me like lava onto the stone-white hospital floors.

I clearly remember confirming with Taylor's pre-surgical nurses that she was allergic to the very antibiotic they nevertheless gave her. Taylor was wearing her red wristband, standard hospital protocol for indicating an allergy. If you're an anesthesiologist, looking for that red wristband is part of your everyday life in the OR. How they missed it, I will never know. What I do know is a simple failure to check her allergies caused Taylor a dangerous complication and would require a second surgery.

I not only questioned the hospital and the anesthesiologist but also God. Hadn't she suffered enough? Why did she have to suffer even more because of human medical error? In one moment, I was angry with God and the next worried that my anger might get in the way of God helping her. Or did it have nothing to do with God? I went to the hospital chapel, as I always did, and lay on the floor crying in front of the altar, kissing the ground. I put my lips to a filthy floor, thinking that somehow punishing myself might help Taylor.

The remainder of the day was a complete blur of joy and relief that Taylor made it through. She was a horror to look at, but she was alive and with us. When Taylor awakened after surgery, she was intubated, attached to a respirator, and unable to speak. But she looked down, saw the writing all over her body, and gave a thumbs-up.

Rules prohibited visitors in the ICU right after her surgery. However, we sneaked in a dear friend of Taylor's, Sandy, a tall and good-looking guy with blond hair, sky-blue eyes, and an extremely kind heart. He cared deeply for Taylor and spent endless hours over the years playing games and entertaining her during her hospital stays. Taylor desperately wanted to communicate with him but couldn't speak. With hand motions she managed to tell Sandy to write on her legs. Barbara, Sandy's mom, a blonde whose glowing tan matched her luminescent heart, sat in the corner with me, our eyes overflowing with tears. Neither of us knew what he wrote, but it made Taylor smile.

Two days after surgery, Jordan decided to take the train from our hometown to New York City to see Tales in the ICU. Taylor was on oxygen, barely able to keep her eyes open, but Jordan rested his head upon hers with a concerned but happy smile. I didn't know him well, and I couldn't understand how he was okay seeing his girlfriend in the ICU, looking like someone on the television show *ER*. I would not have blamed him if he ended things right then and there, but I believe he cared deeply for her from the very start.

Later that day, her friends piled into the ICU, flagrantly disregarding the rules that allowed only two visitors at a time. I told the kids, "Try to be quiet so you don't disturb the other patients," but despite my efforts, it all went to hell when the nurses smelled chicken nuggets.

Taylor was only allowed ice chips until she graduated to liquids and applesauce. Earlier, Taylor had begged, "Jordan, can you get me chicken nuggets?" He thought that was a normal request. What did he know about hospital protocol? I figured by the time he got back, her interest in chicken nuggets would have dissipated, and if she tried them, she wouldn't be able to tolerate them. I had nodded, okay, and Jordan was off and running. I admit I was glad Taylor now had Jordan to run around on her food errands as her palate changed daily—and she was a beast if she didn't have whatever food she wanted when she wanted it.

Due to the allergy debacle, Taylor's second surgery was scheduled for five days later. When we made arrangements to transfer Taylor from Weill Cornell to Columbia to complete her surgery, her doctors at Columbia had warned me, "Find a way to leave Weill Cornell with all her paperwork from her surgery and her stay in the ICU." The problem was that parents were forbidden to see these medical records. Naturally, and to no one's surprise, I arrived at Columbia with all the requisite papers in hand.

The following morning, in her hospital room at Columbia, we were abruptly awakened when a young, dark-haired medical fellow walked in and flicked on a strong iridescent light. We had never met him before. My back stiffened immediately as he unexpectedly told us, "If you proceed with surgery, Taylor could lose her life." I screamed, "Who the hell are you, and what are you talking about?" Taylor turned white as a sheet and began shaking uncontrollably. No one had ever uttered words like this to Taylor before.

Somehow, I found the strength to regain my cool and calmly say, "No worries, T; he doesn't know what he is talking about. I will go find out." She was usually reassured by my words, but this time her eyes bulged with fear, tears rolled down her face, and she turned away, not wanting to show me how upset she was. Her agony swept through my body as I hugged her tightly. I then looked deep into her brown eyes and said in a low whisper, "Listen carefully. Mommy will take care of this. You are not dying." However, the damage was done, and once again Taylor suffered the severe emotional consequences of medical error.

I left the room with the fellow, my face raging. Before he could utter another word, I roared, "How dare you tell my child she might die? We don't know who you are. How are you coming up with this conclusion?" It took many deep breaths and a long time for me to calm down before I was willing to listen to his explanation. He replied, "Based upon the downward trend of her blood numbers, she may not be able to survive surgery." Remember all those papers I brought from Weill Cornell? He had never looked at them, and the fact was her blood numbers were trending upwards. I replied, "You are dead *wrong*!" I couldn't have been held down at this point; I swear I almost lunged at him and threw him down. I had enough strength at that point to lift a car.

I called Bob, and he arrived immediately. The doctors knew they had their hands full with the two of us. Bob entered the room in warrior mode. He didn't even take off his coat or drop his briefcase but instantly became raucous, screaming, "Do you understand the impact your fellow had by telling Sue and Taylor there is a chance she will die? And by the way, Sue knew he was wrong, incompetent, emotionally inept, and twisted. Do you understand what telling someone she could die means? Get him far away from us. If we ever see him again, there will be hell to pay!"

Bob probably could've been heard from 168th Street all the way down to Wall Street. Being married almost twenty-five years at that point, I could count on one hand the number of times Bob lost his temper this dramatically. He was usually calm and cool, but when it involved Taylor's well-being, it was a different story. The doctors knew it was time to buckle up.

Taylor came through the surgery well, and despite all the mishaps along the way, she was now officially in recovery mode.

I reached out to the disciplinary board to take the fellow to task. My goal was to make sure this didn't happen to another child. When I entered the board meeting, all eyes were pointed downward, as if they were children in a principal's office. I politely sat down and explained, "This fellow, whom we had never met before, came into our hospital room unannounced, and his first words were, 'If you proceed with surgery, you may die,' addressing my fifteen-year-old daughter." I glanced at the offending fellow and implored him to fully admit he was wrong. "He is completely incompetent and negligent. I, without any medical background, knew his assumptions were incorrect." I continued reciting the details. The board listened and replied, "We have enough information. You are completely correct, Mrs. Matthews."

Finally, some justice in the medical world! I was satisfied with the hope that no child would have to endure the ineptitude of this doctor. I walked out of the room in what felt like a puff of smoke, vindicated, and moved on. We had bigger fish to fry.

After Taylor was discharged from Columbia, we still needed to go back to Weill Cornell for a post-op consultation with her surgeon. That was when we mentioned our upcoming trip to Great Exuma, scheduled in a few weeks at the end of February.

I will never forget the burning look in her doctor's eyes when he turned to me, clearly disgusted, and shouted, "Are you crazy? You planned a trip to Great Exuma just after a massive thoracotomy? Do you realize they have no medical care and a case of malaria has been reported within the last year?" I glared at him scathingly and, without a hint of hesitation or apology, replied, "Yes, I do." I wanted to say, "And quite frankly, the risks of going to Great Exuma are far smaller than the risks of being in your operating room where my child almost died from anaphylactic shock!"

Glory Be to God Above, She's in Love!

Taylor escaped hospital jail by Valentine's Day, a week before we headed off to Great Exuma. Bob and I had always made sure that our girls didn't consider Valentine's Day a Hallmark holiday, but a day celebrating unconditional love. When the girls were little, they wore Valentine's Day-themed clothes, and our morning tradition was to draw any type of heart they fancied on their faces with my lipstick. Bob always arrived home with magnificent roses for all four of his girls.

On Valentine's Day, and every day, I know I'm blessed that I met the love of my life almost four decades ago. Tragically, a high percentage of couples break up when they lose a child, but our heartbreak has only strengthened our bond. The girls are determined to find men that fit their dad's very large shoes. Andrea, who was only fourteen when we got married, says she too had Bob and me in mind when she was looking for her Mr. Wonderful, and she certainly found him.

As the girls grew up, their own Valentine's Day stories became part of our lives. No matter which one of them had a boyfriend on any particular year, their boyfriends were always invited to join our family rather than going out alone. On Valentine's Day 2007, Taylor and Jordan had been dating for about six weeks. What was he to think?

Mischievous Jordan had a plan that we all knew about except Taylor. With great excitement, he explained, "I'm going to give to someone in each of Taylor's classes a red rose with a clue." We were anxious to hear where the clues would lead, but he never revealed his final intention, if there was one. Nevertheless, his exuberance was contagious.

We awoke on Valentine's Day morning to clean, white, delicate, and perfectly shaped snowflakes blanketing the roads. It was Mother Nature at her finest. Taylor had always been conflicted about Mother Nature. She would often ask, "Mommy, why does Mother Nature create sunsets, rainbows, and calm waters— and also create forest fires, tsunamis, and tornadoes?" I never had an answer, but the beautiful snowstorm on Valentine's Day meant school was closed and Jordan's rose hunt was off. Ryan, Taylor, Corey, and I were huddled under the covers watching reruns of *Full House* on our pullout sofa when the doorbell rang.

Jordan leapt up the steps, grinning, holding a basket overflowing with Valentine's goodies, including a singing card and a bundle of somewhat droopy red roses. I laughed to myself, thinking he probably got them the prior day and didn't put them in water. He climbed into bed next to Taylor with all of us and watched proudly as she unwrapped her gifts. He had an adorable explanation for each one. Taylor immediately snatched his card, not wanting anyone else to read it for obvious reasons.

A Hole Other Problem

It was time for our trip to Great Exuma. Great Exuma is a small island located in the Bahamas that can only be accessed by a small plane. Corey was petrified of small planes, frantic as we waited on the tarmac. As we climbed the narrow stairs leading into the plane, Taylor grabbed her little sister's hand, and they ran to the back of the plane. Snuggled next to each other, they were giggling. I turned my head, smiled to myself, and savored the moment. Years later I found out that Taylor had secretly told Corey, "I'm also scared to fly in this plane." What Corey didn't know at the time was that Taylor was fibbing. Taylor always flew by the seat of her pants, and this time was no different.

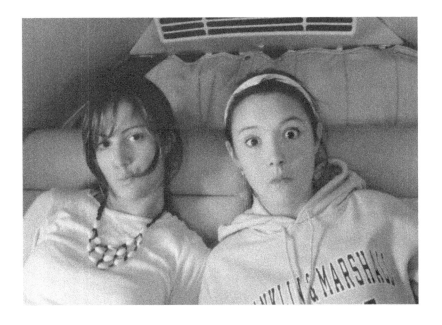

The trip became a whirlwind of teen drama between Taylor and Jordan. They were scheming together to figure out a way for him to sail from his vacation in Florida to Great Exuma. As we sat on the white sand beaches watching the turquoise water roll in, Taylor carried on with Jordan on the phone, "How long do you think it will take to sail here? Can you take your Dad with you? Can you sneak out?" Each morning I went to the front desk and added more minutes to her cell phone as the two lovebirds conspired endlessly. Back-and-forth banter continued all week. Taylor didn't want to take no for an answer.

The girls snorkeled, swam, had massages and pedicures, laughed all night, and watched movies. I reveled in watching Taylor's hair, wispy like the leaves of a palm tree, softly blowing in the wake of an ocean breeze. We were a family united and had left all our medical issues behind. It was not lost on us that just a few weeks earlier, Taylor could have easily died from anaphylaxis during surgery.

Rather abruptly, mid-week through our trip, we noticed a yellowish liquid slowly seeping out of Taylor's mending scars from her surgery. She came to us swearing "I can hear a whooshing sound of air coming from my back when I move." When Tales moved her arms in a rowing motion, the air moved in and out of the hole that had formed at the sight of the last scoliosis incision. We tried to make a joke about it, but funny it certainly was not. I cleaned the area, put her to bed, and remained determined to enjoy our vacation. I thought I had become somewhat invincible when it came to Taylor's medical issues.

The next morning, I froze as I saw Bob's face. Taylor's sheets were covered in liquid. I was certain medical transport back to New York would be needed. As I waited for the on-call doctor to call back, I could feel the blood pulsing through my head; all I could do was frantically throw all of our clothes into bags, readying us to leave on a moment's notice while Ryan and Corey silently watched in horror.

Finally, the phone rang. "Mrs. Matthews, describe exactly what is going on."

Hastily I explained, "A small hole has opened up on Taylor's back along the line of her incision, and a yellowish liquid is seeping out."

"Okay, keep the area clean; get gauze and fill the hole," the doctor instructed.

I implored frantically, "Should I do that while I wait for a med-a-vac back home?"

"Mrs. Matthews, you must have misunderstood. That's not necessary! Enjoy your vacation, and we will see Taylor when you return."

My head was spinning as adrenaline raced through my veins like a rash.

"What? I don't need to bring her to the hospital?"

"No, Mrs. Matthews," he emphatically replied. "Don't come back!"

We spent the remainder of the trip trying to ignore the elephant in the room and enjoy ourselves—doctor's orders. The ocean shimmered against the glow of the sunshine; the softness and warmth of the sand tickled our feet as we soaked up the sunlight. One afternoon I strolled down the beach away from my family and looked back at each imprint my feet had left in the sand, as if I was leaving my mark. As I turned back, I watched my imprints get swept away by the soft, flowing waves.

I stopped at a random place and walked as far back from the ocean as possible, suddenly fearing it. I sat down in the sand, imagining what would happen if I just walked into the ocean until the water consumed me. Would I suffer greatly from drowning? Would I be afraid? Wouldn't it be an easy escape? In some ways, it was tempting. Soon the clouds covered the sun, and the shade rolled in. Somehow my mind snapped back to reality, leaving me totally confused. Why had thoughts about death suddenly infiltrated my thoughts? Could it have been foreshadowing?

It was the last week of February 2007, and we headed back to New York to find out what new turn we'd be taking. Little did we know this would be the beginning of a whole new and foreign chapter in Taylor's odyssey.

The one hole in Taylor's back had turned into two, and both grew so large that I could see Taylor's spine and the scoliosis rods running parallel thereto. I was told to "pack" the holes with sterile gauze dipped in saline solution twice per day. Terrified, I questioned the doctors repeatedly, "How are you going to fix this?" They replied, "For now, let's wait and see." This approach never sat well with us.

We went to MD Anderson for a second opinion. Taylor's oncologists took one look at her back and suggested a consult with a plastic surgeon. Off we went, on golf carts provided by the hospital, across what we called the "city" of MD Anderson. The plastic surgeon, whose face I cannot remember but whose bedside manner repulsed me, carefully examined Taylor and urgently declared, "Taylor's back has to be cut open immediately. She is subject to an infection that could kill her." Corey was with us, only twelve years old at the time. She started to shake as she was about to burst into tears, but then suddenly, Corey became very calm. Unbeknownst to us, Taylor had texted Corey from across the room, "Don't worry, I hear this all the time. It's bullshit."

Until surgery could be scheduled, when the wound was smaller, the plastic surgeon suggested we use a "vac" to keep Taylor's wound clean and safe. A portable vac is a device that is supposed to seal skin together over several weeks or months until surgery can be done. A suction cup that seals itself to the skin, covering the entire wound, is attached to a vacuum machine. The machine must be plugged in to remain charged. If the vac charges all night, the battery can last most of the next day. This was yet another twist that seemed reasonable to the doctors but repugnant and extremely frightful to us.

For this process to be viable, I—a CPA by trade, not a nurse practitioner—had to remove the bandages and sponge every other night, exposing a large, cavernous hole that resembled a piece of raw, red steak the size of a large lemon on my own daughter's back, and replace the bandages. Even this veteran mom was not up for that task!

When Taylor objected to the idea, the doctor dug his piercing eyes into Taylor's, without regard for the fact that he was speaking to a fifteen-year-old, and in a threatening tone implored, "You're risking your life if you don't comply." We were startled and angry at his dictatorial tone. We didn't go for browbeating Tales, and we certainly never scared her into treatment options. But this time she had no choice but to acquiesce.

Hooking Taylor up to the vac resulted in a colossal surge of compression that was extremely painful. I had to place my emotions somewhere far in the distance to be able to inflict such pain on my daughter. Taylor didn't complain, but the tears dripping off her newly grown eyelashes told the whole story. The healing process, if it worked on such a large area, could take up to a year. This was not an option for us. Again, the search for new doctors began. This time they were plastic surgeons. Quite a different experience!

A sure way to raise Taylor's spirits, as well as Ryan's and Corey's, was a visit to London to visit Aunt Andrea and her family. Earlier that year, Andrea had given birth to her second baby girl, Sofia Rose. She was an angel brought to us from heaven on fairy wings. Although she was born under the rainy London sky, Sofia was cloaked in sunshine from the minute she looked at her mommy with her enormous dark-brown eyes.

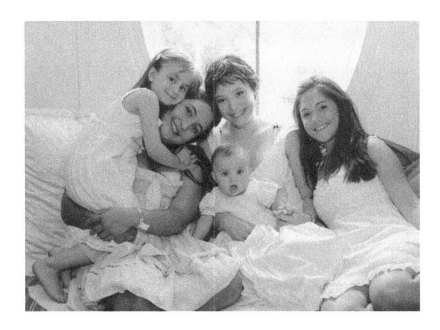

As an only child, when Samantha found out she was going to have a sibling, she was none too pleased. Andrea explained that God had sent them a new baby. That actually wasn't too far off; after several miscarriages, they didn't think they could have another child. Then Bill had a vivid dream—a message from God— that they should try again, and that time their prayers were answered.

After contemplating the news for a few seconds, she turned to Andrea and asked, with hands on hips, "Can we email God and tell him we don't want a new baby?"

"If only, Samantha, we could access God through email and ask him for favors!" was all Andrea could muster before she broke out into laughter.

Eager to meet Sofia, we confidently planned an Easter trip overseas, vac and all! The doctors argued, "A cross-Atlantic trip is impossible!" They added, with gravity, "The battery pack might not last all the way to London; the vac can't be turned off for more than two hours before Taylor will be at serious risk of getting an infection." Ignoring the doctor's skepticism, we were more worried by the need to use an electric power adaptor for the unit while in London. If you've ever burned out a hair dryer or electric appliance while using a converter, you can imagine our concern.

The obstacles were becoming insurmountable—time for Bob to take charge. He ascertained that a global company made the vac, and they had a London location. The Brits were only too happy to rent us a unit built for the UK and deliver it right to Aunt Annie's flat. The trip was back on.

Just then, my mother took a turn for the worse. She had been sick for four years, almost the same amount of time as Taylor, with emphysema. As the years passed, my mom's breathing got worse, and her anxiety understandably became extreme. With each passing month, her home looked like ours, filled with medical equipment and prescription bottles.

In April 2007, my mom was placed in the hospital, and she chose to enroll in hospice. She wasn't panicked but a bit melancholy, which was uncharacteristic of her. During one of Andrea's last conversations with her by phone, she soothingly explained, "Don't worry, Andrea. I love you now, and I'll love you a thousand years from now." Was that the beginning of a goodbye? We weren't sure. Andrea was reluctant to fly overseas because Sofia was an infant, barely three months old, but in the end we decided to reverse course. Instead of traveling to London for Easter, Andrea's family came to New York to see my mom for the last time.

My mom died on Friday the thirteenth—not a surprise as she was born on April Fools' Day. Her birthday and the day she left us together form a metaphor for how she lived her life: always witty, capricious, and on the edge. She was truly a character, someone who lived to "stir the pot" and always had to have the last word, similar to my sister Lynn. She died peacefully, surrounded by family. In the corner, snuggled in a warm blanket, lay beautiful little Sofia, who we had all just met for the first time only days prior.

Following my mom's funeral, my father brought us all back to the house and hastily gave us the jewelry she left for each of us. We each were given a small wooden box, the type you would see at a garage sale (atypical of my mom), which held an index card detailing what she had left for each of her children and granddaughters. The cards were written in my dad's precise, all-upper-case handwriting. The room went silent. I thought, *Rita, what were you thinking when you had Daddy cross out and add items to the cards?* My mom's most precious charm bracelet, where every special memory in her life was etched in fourteen-carat gold, had been deleted on one card and added to mine. Diamond earrings were similarly transferred from one sibling to another. It all seemed so random. Was this an April Fool's joke? *Really, Dad, couldn't you have rewritten the index cards?*

Years later, I realized the cards were probably purposely not rewritten. In true Rita form, she wanted us to know that sometimes we were in her good graces and other times we were not. Most important, she wanted to have the last word!

The Great Escape

It turned out the vac never did work completely. Once again, Taylor and I returned to the surgical suite. This time, a reconstructive plastic surgeon would open her wound and stretch muscle and connective tissue into the space, secure it in place, and then connect the skin over it. His work was masterful.

At the same time, fluid was accumulating in Taylor's lungs. We pushed Interventional Radiology at Columbia to drain it, but for a reason unbeknownst to us, they repeatedly refused.

On April 26, thirteen days after we lost my mom, Tales developed a high fever. We rushed her to the Columbia emergency room where they confirmed that the fluid in Taylor's lungs was infected. They still declined to drain it.

After some rather ugly conversations with the staff and a seemingly eternal wait, I became irate, demanding a discharge to take Tales to a hospital that would drain the fluid. The ER doctors threatened to call security, physically restrain me, handcuff me, and take me to jail. Apparently, in New York State, after you have admitted a child, you can be prevented from removing her if the hospital thinks her life is in jeopardy. I was astounded that the doctors refused to intervene to save her life and simultaneously wouldn't allow us to leave.

Tales watched from afar as my argument with the ER doctor escalated. She had become immune to my tantrums, and she knew no matter what the situation, Bob and I would take care of it. With a roll of her eyes, she tossed her hand and flippantly declared, "I can't deal with all the drama. I'm going to sleep." I walked around the ER, black eyes darting from corner to corner, trying to determine if we could escape unnoticed. The Columbia emergency room, like most inner-city hospitals, was jammed full of true emergencies as well as oddball needs that had been pushed aside until the wee hours of the night. This night was as bad as any, but the nurses kept their eyes glued on me. There was no escaping.

Huddled in the corner of a filthy ER bathroom for privacy, I called Bob. Tears began pooling slowly and then fell all at once, like a soft drizzle that unexpectedly erupts into a storm. "They refuse to drain Taylor's lungs, and the fluid is infected! And I confirmed with the doctor on call, there is a high likelihood Taylor could die if her lungs aren't drained." Bob was furious and horrified but said with confidence, "I'm on it." In the middle of the night, he turned to a familiar source of counsel.

As far back as our first days at Sloan, Bob's friend Dr. Len Girardi had been offering help. Len is one of the most talented and successful heart surgeons in the world and the chair of Weill Cornell's department of cardiothoracic surgery. Bob called him at home and asked if he could get Tales to Weill Cornell. He didn't hesitate for a second. Len suggested we check ourselves out and drive immediately downtown. When Bob told him we were being prohibited from leaving, he attempted to work it out with the ER doctor. To his shock, the ER doctor refused. Not to be denied, Len arranged for an ambulance transfer to Weill Cornell, the only way Columbia would permit us to leave.

I awakened Taylor, and as we walked outside, it felt like a release from prison. The blinking red lights of the awaiting ambulance enveloped me as if they were emanating from a beautiful sunrise. A new day was dawning—a day in which Taylor would escape death. In a sleepy, dreamy state, Taylor looked into my eyes for just a second, then put her hand into mine and mouthed, "Thank you," as my emotions soared. Len admitted us directly to his intensive care unit at Weill Cornell to avoid the ER and pediatrics. By early the next morning, Weill Cornell Interventional Radiology drained Taylor's lungs, by way of a sonogram, without issue.

Once again, her survival came down to different doctors, different hospitals, and different solutions.

Where Every Day Is Magical

I remember Taylor's words as if they were spoken yesterday: "Mommy, can I plan a Make-a-Wish trip to Disney World?" Remember, a few years back Make a Wish had backed out of Taylor's over-the-top tree house wish, leaving her still with one magic wish. I laughed out loud. "Really? Disney World at fifteen years old? Are you serious, Tales?"

"Yesssss, Mommy! And I want Ryan, Corey, and all my friends to come, too!" Now it made more sense. Like a volcano, and with her typically heightened level of exuberance, she spewed out the names of all the friends she wanted to invite. "Okaayyy?" she insisted impatiently, wanting an immediate answer. Quickly, I mentally calculated the numbers and arrived at a startling party of *ten* teenagers, with only Bob and I as chaperones. I would have to dig deep and head into "super mom" mode for this one. "Okay, little T," I said, with smiling eyes.

I let my memory drift to the last time we were in Disney World, four weeks prior to Taylor's diagnosis. While in Epcot Center, we participated in a special program called Leave Your Legacy. Our photo was taken, and we were told it would be mounted onto a steel plate, engraved, and permanently adhered to a stone in Disney World. Several weeks later, we received a copy of the steel plates in the mail. Taylor looked at her picture, bellowing, "Ewww, I look bald!" Her hair was pulled back in a tight ponytail. The irony sends chills spiraling throughout my body. The program has since been discontinued, but it comforts me to know that concrete evidence of our family of five is etched in stone at the happiest place on earth.

A lovely, petite blonde from Make a Wish, face aglow with hope and energy, arrived at our doorstep, eager to plan a trip to Disney for our family. Unlike the tree house, this kind of wish was easy for them. Little did they know that we were also planning on taking seven of Taylor's friends!

Taylor asked, "Where will we be staying?"

"The Make a Wish Hotel; it's about ten miles from the entrance to Disney World." Out of respect, Taylor tried to hold it together, merely nodding her head, while fully comprehending that staying there meant other sick children would surround her, the last thing she wanted.

I winked at Taylor, and immediately her composure and playful smile returned. She knew I was on her team, her partner in crime and a master in the art in getting things done our way. Instead of their hotel, we ended up booking rooms at the Boardwalk Inn and got Make a Wish to agree. We never told them about the other kids.

The days leading up to the trip were filled with joyous moments. One afternoon Tales returned from shopping with Jordan and shrieked, "Mommy, look what I bought!" Out came bright white sneakers with yellow shoelaces. That seemed reasonable until, in one swift motion, she turned them over and out popped orange rollers from underneath. She saw the look of bewilderment on my face and immediately explained, "Mommy, now I will be able to keep up with my friends because I have sneakers that roll like skates." Reality stung, like a bad bee bite. Taylor's lung capacity was below 50 percent at this point, but she didn't want to tell any of her friends.

The day before we left, Jordan arrived holding a bag full of white hats, each embroidered with "Tay" in bright orange, for everyone on the trip. It seemed like an adorable idea at the time. When we arrived at the airport, in two shiny, extra-long limos, the excitement was overflowing, like perspiration after a long run.

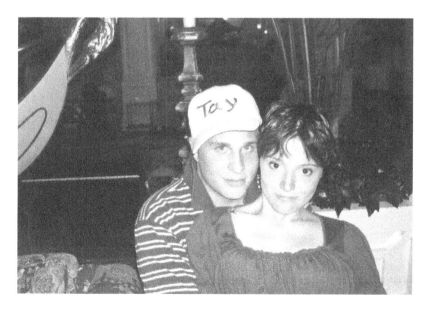

We arrived at the Boardwalk Inn, located on the Disney Boardwalk, which, with its carnival games and electrifying nightlife, had the decadence of old-world Atlantic City. The buildings are multicolored, with pastel façades set against bright, flashing signs that implored you to come their way. It was a sensory feast.

As everyone settled in, Bob and I went to the Make a Wish compound to get what turned out to be the best gift of all: fast passes entitling us to skip all the lines! The hotel reminded us of the hospital. I looked at all the children with sorrow, thinking, "These are their last wishes." It literally never crossed my mind that Taylor, too, could be terminal. I was fully aware of how compromised Taylor was, but she was so full of excitement, planning her life, it seemed nothing could stop her. She was eager to go back to school, had signed up to take the SATs, and had begun considering where she wanted to go to college. I was in an "accidentally on purpose" state of denial, refusing to let my brain acknowledge the worst, but I think she truly thought the world was still her oyster.

Back at the hotel, we delightfully listened to uproarious laughter emanating from the kids' rooms. I entered their rooms, and it appeared as if they had been hit by a Disney World tornado; the kids looked like a bunch of overgrown six-year-olds amidst a sea of Mickey, Minnie, Donald, and all the princesses.

Bob and I were in full-on work mode, coordinating meeting times, handing out water bottles, and issuing and collecting park passes, all the while finding restaurants for parties of twelve. We left the hotel each day at the crack of noon. We were, after all, on teenage time. It was ninety-eight degrees every day, with 90 percent humidity. If it hadn't been for the special passes, there is little doubt we would have left a trail of teenagers and two overheated, stressed-out parents passed out along Main Street USA.

Jordan helped Taylor go up and down the small hills of the park with her "roller-sneakers." Ryan and Corey were close by to help. At one point, Ryan intervened by carrying Taylor on her back, and then we rented a Disney stroller. Taylor was a sight to be seen in the stroller, but she didn't care. Every day, in addition to her "Tay" hat, she adorned a massive grin.

Meanwhile, many of Taylor's friends thought she was blowing them off in favor of Jordan and arrogantly ran ahead. With tears saturating her shirt, she asked, "Mommy, how can I tell them I can't keep up with their pace? And why won't my friends wear the Tay hats?" I had no answer. However, it was as clear as a crystal ball that they were sending a message. They were rejecting Jordan and his hats.

We stumbled upon the legendary Beaches and Cream ice cream parlor. Their signature dessert, "The Kitchen Sink," consisted of a mammoth bowl of ice cream overflowing with sugar-charged treats. To be exact, the dessert contains twenty-eight different ingredients, including many flavors of ice cream, syrups, toppings, brownies, cookies, and more, and is nothing short of a frosty bowl of pure gluttony.

As the others ordered a single scoop of ice cream or a brownie, Jordan, playing the role of the court jester, geared up for the feast. The main lights dimmed and other lights flashed as the Kitchen Sink was being delivered. Only at Disney World would there be major pomp and circumstance surrounding a dessert. The contest began, whereby if someone can eat the entire dessert in a prescribed amount of time, they win an enormous prize. With rolled-up sleeves and determination in his eyes, Jordan dug in. We watched him with both awe and disgust. Jordan tried as hard as he could, at first rapidly scarfing down the confection with gusto, until he slowed down and could barely take another bite. He didn't give up, eating until the buzzer rang, at which point he lost. Worse yet, he immediately ran out of the restaurant and vomited profusely, but even that didn't quell our laughter.

While in Epcot, we heard the booming sound of what we knew had to be fireworks. We ran out of where we were eating dinner to watch the dancing colors illuminating the sky. Jordan took Taylor aside and wrapped his hands around her waist as she leaned against him. I could see the flicker in her eyes and the warmth they exchanged. Taylor later told me, with a dreamy expression, "It was magical, Mommy."

The next night, I caught on that Jordan had been sleeping in Taylor's bed with her, in the same room shared with her friends. Now some of the puzzle made sense. I could better understand why some of the girls left Taylor behind and were angry with Jordan. It was supposed to be an all-girls sleepover. I insisted that Jordan return to his room permanently.

My mind drifted back to the good old days when the girls were little and they used to have play dates. Taylor could always persuade her friends to join in with her antics. Her friend Allie wrote in the school newsletter, "She was super friendly, and we became fast friends. Taylor could make a friend in a heartbeat. I never knew how she did it. After spending five minutes, they would have a substantial connection with her. Taylor's energy and fearlessness were enormously contagious."

As the kids giggled over the breakfast menu, going back and forth on whether they should get Mickey or Minnie pancakes, Bob and I were sad. The Jordan drama was escalating, and the group was becoming erratic. We both knew Taylor didn't have the energy at this point to handle it. I explained to the girls that Jordan was helping Taylor because, "Taylor has never wanted you to know her lung condition or how sick she really is." I think they thought I was fibbing. For over four years, Tales had successfully hidden from her friends the extent of her illness. I guess they couldn't or didn't want to comprehend the truth.

At the same time, plenty of fun abounded. One morning, Make a Wish organized a breakfast with the Disney characters. At fifteen, the kids engaged with the characters as if they were young tykes. Another day, they went into a store and squeezed themselves into princess costumes made for much younger kids, laughing until they cried. I guess the magic of Disney really does exist, transforming people of any age into their younger alter egos. Fast forward ten hours, and the kids were ready to act *older* than their ages. As we crossed the glimmering half-moon entrance into Pleasure Island, full of noise, crowds, and clubs, the kids were eager to party into the night, and that's just what they did.

When we returned home from Disney, we immediately jumped into full-fledged panic mode to get Ryan ready to leave for her freshman year at Wake Forest. As a small liberal arts college with Division I athletic sports, it is the perfect mixture of a great education with a "rah rah" mentality. We were so incredibly proud of her. Not only did she handle the SATs and applications basically on her own, but Wake was also her first choice, and she made it happen. It's hard to ask for more, but she gave us more: she was following her dreams but never lost sight of the importance of her family.

Ryan was nervous about leaving home and felt it was a breaking point in her life. She told me later, "In my mind this signaled the last time things would ever be the same again, the last time we would all live together as a family. I didn't want to be alone any more than I already was, and I didn't want to lose my family. I was holding on with a death grip. I kind of hate remembering that girl. But in true me form, I knew I was supposed to go to college and be excited, and I wanted to pretend I was normal, or at least have other people believe it, so I just kept moving. Part autopilot, part coping mechanism, part denial."

Corey didn't have a good understanding of what it would feel like when Ryan left home for college. "There are a lot of things I could have and should have been more sensitive about when it came to Ryan's milestones, and this was one of them. I don't think I knew how sad I would feel about Ryan leaving until we got in the car to go to the airport, only two of us in the backseat instead of three."

Taylor felt the same way. She made the best of it, telling Corey, "Don't worry; we'll have fun," and she meant it, but a piece of Taylor's heart broke off and went to Wake Forest that day with her big sister.

It was heartbreaking to say goodbye to Ryan, even though as parents we do our best to embrace our children's milestones, and we knew it was time to give Ryan her wings to soar. We returned home to now another "new normal."

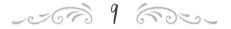

9

Learning to Fly

Sunshine mixed with a little hurricane.

–Anonymous

The A School

Tales was in school almost full-time for the first time in ages. She was particularly excited, as she had been accepted into Edgemont High School's Alternative School, known as "the A School," beginning her junior year.

The A School allows students to learn independently in an open and non-judgmental environment, fostering independence in life and education. In Taylor's interview, her teachers Pam and Cory (students were allowed to use first names to address their teachers) told me, "Taylor didn't want to be 'the kid with cancer' anymore and was seeking a new label, a new community to be a part of, a place where she could truly be herself."

The A School is located in a separate section of the high school, with a private ingress and egress, and is filled with bright paintings, posters, and comfy leather couches covered with graffiti. When I first visited, the room itself invited me in, persuading me to find peace and comfort in its four walls. I could see why Taylor loved it there. I laughed to myself as my eyes perused the writing on the couches. Students finally got to write all over the furniture, something most three-year-olds crave (and are punished for), and now it was not only allowed but also encouraged. Taylor adored the idea of working in a comfortable environment where thinking outside the box was applauded. Despite its uncharacteristic appearance, it's definitely a place that whets one's appetite for knowledge.

While lying across one of the leather couches, Taylor exclaimed, "I can't believe I'm here. Pam, how lucky am I?" Pam responded, "Actually, we're the lucky ones, because we have you here." It was the first time in over four years that Taylor found a place where she fit in and where she felt comfortable talking about her illness. Taylor's other beloved and talented A School teacher, Cory, gave me a poem Taylor wrote about the A School, illustrating her warm feelings of acceptance:

The Different One
I was the only red bird in the entire nest.
It was hard being the only one, different from all the rest.
Mama said I was lovely, Papa said I was unique,
But all the other little birds–well, they just called me a geek.

As I grew older and I lived a few seasons,
I decided I had to go out and find the reason.

I told Mama and Papa I needed to see the wise mouse,
The mouse that lived up in the tiny tree house.

So off I went wandering and soon I was there.
I knocked on his door and took a deep breath of air.

The old wise mouse invited me in
And sat me down so we could begin.

"What is wrong, my beautiful bird?" the old mouse said.
I looked at him and asked, "Well, don't you see, I'm ALL RED!"

"Oh, my sad little bird, you are more beautiful than you can see,
But you think you're different; is that why you have come to see me?"

"Yes, wise old mouse, and what do I do?
The only person I thought could help me was you!"

"Oh, little one, I cannot change your color,
But even if I could, I would not make you any duller."
I was shocked and sad; I could not believe it was true.
But the wise mouse said one other thing I think you should know, too.
He told me, "You must learn to love who you are,
Then you will find that you can be a star."

I flew from his house so sad and confused
That I took the wrong path, not the one I should have used.

I flew for an hour until it began to get dark.
I was scared and tired but I found a little tiny park.

I perched in the tree and began to count my sheep,
And sooner or later I fell fast asleep.

I dreamed of a place where no one would make fun,
A place where I would fit in with everyone.

I woke in the morning to a loud ringing bell.
And what happened next, I'm so excited to tell.

Well, I searched for my food and I sat in my tree
And I watched a teacher drink her morning tea.

Kids of all types entered a small school
And I noticed that not one kid was ever cruel.

The teacher spoke of what their school was about.
It sounded so great I wanted to shout!

I flew towards the window to hear more
And what I heard made my heart soar.

I flew through a gap
And found my way to Cory's lap.

For this was the A School
And I had no doubt that these kids were cool.

Though Cory screamed and shooed me off,
Nick caught me and got everyone's attention with a cough.

"This bird is special; she's not the same.
Don't you see she's as red as a flame?"

They took a vote as A-Schoolers do
And they decided that I could stay with them, too.

So this is my story, and why I am here today
To tell you all how happy I am that I could stay.

The A School is a wonderful place
And a family like them I could never replace.

I'm happy you are here to listen to my story
And I never could have written it without you, Cory.

Tales was stubborn, strong minded, and determined to engage in all A School activities, including a fall overnight camping trip. When deciding what to allow Taylor to do, Bob and I always considered her doctors' advice while weighing the risks against the rewards of living life, but ultimately, we went with our instincts. I imagine I asked all the right questions: "Is there medical care nearby? Who will be keeping an eye on Taylor?" However, I don't remember the answers, and I'm not sure I cared. She was adamant that she was going on the trip regardless of what her doctors said, uninterested in her physical limitations. She gloried in the fact that her teachers wanted her to go. What Bob and I had to say mattered very little.

In the end, Taylor muscled her way into getting her way. She went on the trip and participated in every activity, even those strictly forbidden by her doctors, including scaling a mountain, crossing a tightrope, and running through the woods. She was gushing with stories, including those about hikes that had become treks through ten-foot reeds. Taylor truly felt normal and part of the A School family so much that she didn't even seem to mind at all that she returned home completely covered in poison ivy.

Houston, We Have a Problem

That fall we headed back to MD Anderson in search of answers. We knew the tumors were still growing, and one tumor was particularly threatening because its position made it almost impossible to operate on. While we certainly were used to hospitals by now, it never got any easier. As we sat in a humorless, bright-yellow waiting room, staring at walls covered in children's artwork, juxtaposed against fear, dread, and the stench of heartbreak, my mind raced as I held back tears. I attempted to breathe, looking across the room into another mother's eyes, understanding like no one else could the extent of her pain. At the same time, as each mother also understood, we had to paint bright smiles on our faces for the sake of our children. My constant chorus was, "Don't worry, sweet baby; Mommy and Daddy will make it all better."

After an exhausting but productive Monday in Houston, we flew home Tuesday morning, waiting to hear the doctor's suggestions. As soon as we stepped foot in our home, the fun-loving, energetic, spirited Taylor came out to play. She was full of piss and vinegar, as my dad would say. This particular Tuesday was no different, and I remember breathing a momentary sigh of relief as Corey took me into her loving arms and said, "Mommy, I'm so happy you guys are home!" Corey's soft, rosy cheeks became one with my own, as she held me tightly and I took in her scent. My baby.

On Wednesday morning, soon after dropping the girls off at school, the call arrived. "We think Taylor needs a specialized type of radiation. Can you fly back to Houston this afternoon to do the molds?"

"What are molds?"

"To target Taylor's tumor for radiation therapy, molds are used to hold her body as still as possible," the doctor calmly explained. The radiation chosen was IMRT, a very precise radiation that attempts to kill tumors without harming nearby tissue. Bob had been discussing IMRT and Proton Beam Radiation for years with anyone who would listen. Now they agreed.

My body shook. Were they kidding me? We had just been in Texas the past two days. It broke my heart to even think about telling Corey that Mommy was leaving yet again. Corey was on her own, at twelve years old, because Ryan was at college. I had to look into her eyes and tell her to be strong, because once again we were leaving.

Naturally, Corey was heartbroken. At the same time, this had been her life for the last four years, so it was, in some ways, her reality. That didn't make it any easier, only more tragic. The worst part was I had to go; there was no ability to compromise. With a heavy heart, on Wednesday afternoon, we made our way back to Houston. The doctors completed the radiation molds, and we flew back to New York on Thursday.

How did I manage to fly Taylor back and forth from New York to Houston twice that week, knowing we would return to Houston just three days later on Sunday to begin treatment on Monday morning? We had already clocked 5,700 air miles for the week.

Sunday night, Taylor threw a full-blown temper tantrum. She was enraged, kicking and hollering, flailing her arms, entirely unwilling to let go of Jordan. "NO, MOMMY, I am *not* going! I'm so tired and pissed. I want to stay here. I am

NOT GOING to Houston!" She held Jordan tightly and wept. Bob and I gently pried them apart, suppressing the pain in our own hearts. She was inconsolable.

On Monday morning, her radiation oncologist, a charming, kind, and understanding man with whom Taylor instantly bonded, handed Taylor her radiation schedule—every day at two o'clock, Monday through Friday, for four weeks. Suddenly, Taylor's eyes welled with tears. Confused, I asked, "What's up?" Within seconds, Taylor had mentally calculated that the last day of radiation was on November 1, her sixteenth birthday. The number of radiation treatments was not negotiable, and Taylor knew it. I thought, *How in God's name could this have happened?* I wanted to scream, but instead I silently cried.

It didn't take long for our goal-oriented Taylor to figure out a plan. She asked, "Can I have two doses of radiation on the same day?" Her doctor was surprised but eventually chuckled, succumbing to Taylor's uncanny ability to convince most people to see things her way. He was very forthcoming: "Taylor, you will be very sick if you do double radiation in one day, but I will do it."

I thought to myself, *Okay, we'll be home for her birthday; that's great, but I also know she'll never accept missing Halloween, the day before.* I wondered how she would finagle this one! Surprisingly, days passed, and she didn't say anything about it.

Without a word to me, she negotiated with the radiation staff to have radiation at four o'clock instead of two o'clock on Mondays, allowing her to stay home Sunday nights in New York. Additionally, she negotiated a very early time on Friday mornings, so she could fly home early enough to go out Friday nights with her friends. Six nights in Houston magically turned to four, resulting in three nights home each week for the four weeks. I never asked her how she accomplished this, as radiation treatment is set for the same time every day.

Taylor was on the path to advocating for herself and taking control of her own life. We had a fair amount of experience, so when the doctors said, "Jump," we had the courage to ask for better answers or even to simply say no. Many times, that proved to be the right decision. We learned the hard way that there is no way to survive a pediatric cancer diagnosis without being a tenacious, tough, unyielding, and vigorous advocate. You cannot be at the mercy of the doctors or the medical system as it stands today.

Most nights in Houston, we lay in bed, talking and chuckling about anything and everything. Never once did we turn on the TV. It seemed we never ran out of things to talk about. When Taylor felt well, we looked for things to do. We learned one of the biggest tourist attractions in Houston is the mall. Neither of us were fervent shoppers, but "The Houston Mall" promised much more entertainment value than shopping alone.

"Mommy," Taylor read, somewhat tongue in cheek, "listen to this one! This mall, aka the Galleria, attracts 'more than twenty-six million visitors each year who seek the dynamic and fine shopping environment uniquely offered by Texas's largest shopping center.' And get this," she giggled, "they say, 'International guests and Houstonians blend seamlessly in the center. The Galleria is Houston's most popular retail and tourist destination, meeting every style and taste.'" That was enough to get us to belly laugh. We had been in Texas long enough to know that this outing could prove hilarious, especially for two exhausted New Yorkers who were cooped up and nothing short of slap-happy.

We arrived at the Galleria ready for people watching. I know this is a gross generalization, and as a native New Yorker I'm used to being on the receiving end of stereotyping, but as we watched, we couldn't figure out how the shoppers tried on clothes. Their makeup was as thick as caulk, making every wrinkle seem that much deeper; jewelry dripped off them like a leaky faucet, and their jeans, boots, and belts were appropriate for women fifteen years younger and two sizes smaller. How could they endure undressing to buy more?

Taylor and I sat side by side on a wooden bench, hunched together, giggling. Fidgeting, Taylor asked, "When are they coming out? Mommy, how many clothes can they try on?" Eventually, people appeared with enormous treat bags overflowing with bejeweled outfits just "purrrfect" for their next occasion. Most came out without a bleached-blonde hair out of place, although we did catch a few looking a little less than well-coiffed, hot and bothered, leaving their dressing rooms in a hurry. Taylor and I guffawed, tears streaming from our eyes, in hysteria. In the end, our trips to the mall lent themselves to good-hearted amusement when laughter was, indeed, the best and only medicine. It was the relief we needed and, in fact, quite literally craved.

One night we were interrupted by the shuffling and crunching sound of paper being shoved under our hotel door. Taylor knew this meant math homework. Schoolwork was sent to us on numerous occasions over the years, but this time, the papers kept coming and coming. She felt like she was under siege. Before I had a chance to react, Taylor jumped up, grabbed the papers, threw them in the air like a whirling dervish, and screamed, "Fuck her!" (As in, her teacher.) As I watched the papers cascading down onto the floor, I caught Taylor's contagious laughter. I knew that was the end of math homework for a good long time.

When your child throws her homework onto the floor and screams profanities, typically it would be worthy of discussion and punishment. But our mantra had become "anything goes." In many respects, our lives could be summed up by the acronym "SNAFU," coined by the military, meaning, "situation normal: all fucked up," although actually very little about our situation was normal.

About two weeks into treatment, Tales bounced out of the treatment room like a hot air balloon. Jumping over toys, she ran to me shouting, "Mommy, I worked it out! I'm going home for Halloween!" I was filled with excitement, although I was sure her doctors would not allow her to miss her last day of treatment. She could hardly get the words out: "I investigated flights back to New York and found a seven-thirty flight, which will get me home in time for the last period of school!"

"But clinic doesn't even open till eight," I responded, perplexed.

"Mommy, the nurses are coming in at six to give me my last radiation treatment."

Now I was even more confounded. The nurses were only allowed to work eight-hour shifts, typically eight in the morning to four in the afternoon. Their schedules were set, every day, the same as the day before.

"Wait, does that mean they changed their schedules for their other patients?"

"Yes, Mommy!" Taylor roared.

She had solved her Halloween dilemma. I know it gave the nurses great happiness to see the joy they brought to one young girl by helping her make it home for Halloween.

Dear Cancer Girl

One weekend, halfway through treatment, Taylor and I flew from Houston to Ryan's freshman year parents' weekend at Wake. Bob was meeting us there, but unfortunately Corey was back in New York, attending her then best friend's Bat Mitzvah. This was such a special and important weekend for Bob and me. We wanted to be able to enjoy every minute with Ryan. As our plane descended, Taylor's eyes were sparkling with anticipation. She was raring to go, despite a particularly grueling week of radiation.

We headed toward campus, our steps quickening as we approached Ryan's dorm. In Ryan's loving arms, Taylor squeezed her eyes shut, soaking up the warmth and love of her sister.

At dinner Taylor's eyes never left Ryan's, words spilling out like an overflowing river. Taylor hung on to Ryan's every word, constantly imploring, "Tell me more!" Bob and I watched from a distance, as the girls found each other again after worlds apart. They had missed each other desperately.

We returned to the hotel with a peaceful feeling, proud of the connection between our daughters and ecstatic about Ryan's accomplishments thus far. We were excited to tailgate the next day before a Wake Forest football game. Bob fell into a deep slumber as Taylor and I stayed up chitchatting like college students. "Oh, Tales, I forgot to tell you," I said, handing her an envelope, "Daddy brought you mail from home." Snail mail was always an unexpected treat in the world of emails and texts.

As she read, her eyes became wide with a mixture of fear and fury. Her shoulders hunched forward as if something had suddenly jumped upon her back. She gasped and jetted out of the room, slamming the door. I was wildly confused. When she came back, she was a mere fraction of the person she had been at dinner that night, completely overwrought, her beautiful face streaming with thick, salty tears, her hands shaking.

"Taylor, what is going on?" I asked.

"Mommy," she asked in between sobs, "do you think Jordan would ever cheat on me?"

"Of course not, love bug; why?" I breathed a sigh of relief, thinking it was just teenage drama. Blurry eyed, she handed me the letter.

The letter read:

Dear Cancer Girl,
Stay in Houston. It is easier to hook up with Jordan that way.

It was written with letters cut from a magazine. I was in shock. I couldn't fathom the cruelty someone could purposefully inflict on my little girl who was already in such a weak and vulnerable place. The part about Jordan cheating on Taylor was a boldfaced lie, but the salutation was nothing short of wicked.

"How could anyone ever write this to me? And it's someone from home because I saw the postmark."

Taylor sobbed all night. The long-term impact of receiving this letter left a permanent scar, one that cut deeper than any physical wound.

One reason Taylor was bullied is the bully thought her victim wouldn't retaliate, but she underestimated Taylor. She never allowed herself to be a victim. Bad things might happen, but Taylor sized up each one, even cancer, and fought back. Taylor immediately asked that I call a dear friend who was a private investigator. She wanted the girl identified. She wanted to confront her, forcing her to face her acts without the cowardly veil of anonymity. We dissuaded her, as it would only cause more turmoil. She and I did our best to deduce the source, and we ultimately had a pretty good guess as to who wrote the letter.

Taylor slept restlessly that night, but she was able to compartmentalize things, a key to survival. She would let nothing stand in the way of her weekend with her big sister. The next morning, as we approached the stadium parking lot, we saw the asphalt covered in a sea of people boasting Wake Forest colors of black and gold. Winston-Salem is the hometown of the famous Krispy Kreme donuts, which were everywhere, along with wine, beer, and Bloody Mary's served poorly disguised in Wake Forest tumblers.

The team and the fans were hungry for a win! We joined in, chanting, "Go, Demon Deacons!" When there was a play in favor of the "Deacs," the stadium roared in waves of black and gold. It was a sight to be seen, and the icing on the cake was that Wake won the game, resulting in the students streaming rolls of toilet paper onto the trees in the quad, until the green leaves of every tree were merely specks on a sea of white. Needless to say, Taylor was keyed up.

When the time came to say goodbye, Ryan melted in our arms. I can still see Ryan's face as she waved at us until we could no longer see her. Taylor and I waited on the steps of the chapel for our taxi. No words were spoken. She moved closer and cuddled in my arms as her head dropped and tears cascaded down her cheeks. My eyes stung with pungent tears as the lump in my throat swelled. I knew her thoughts were back to "Dear Cancer Girl."

When we got back to Houston, Taylor was ready to start her own college search, and being at MD Anderson didn't stop her. We planned a visit to Rice University in Houston. Before our visit, I suggested to Taylor, "Should you wear something that hides your radiation tattoos?" These were small dots to guide the radiation precisely. She replied, "No, Mommy, I am who I am."

During the information session, Taylor was intrigued by the story of William Rice, the founder of Rice University. Apparently, William's butler, in an attempt to steal a significant amount of money set aside for the university, tried to murder him. The attempt was unsuccessful. Taylor equated the story to her favorite game, Clue. Throughout the school tour, Taylor was in stitches, saying, "It was the butler, in the master bedroom, with the cash."

Let's Get Potato Skins

Still in Houston, Taylor planned a spa day in anticipation of her sixteenth birthday. I knew it was a gift for me more than her. Two years shy of the required age of eighteen, she somehow convinced the spa to allow her in. I was thrilled, but at the same time I couldn't quiet the nagging question in the back of my mind: *Would she ever have a real eighteenth birthday?* I silently begged God for many more birthdays.

She chose our treatments and ordered a full plate of greens, delicately arranged on a white porcelain plate, and my favorite, lemon water. The aroma of the flavors intoxicated me. She attended to every detail to deliver me a perfect day. We luxuriated in soft, white, plush robes, sitting side-by-side and chatting. Taylor's big brown eyes shimmered, glowing with pride and joy in having done something to make me happy.

Before Taylor's last week of treatment, we had a scheduled last appointment with Dr. Anderson. We all loved his bedside manner, admired his brilliance, and were appreciative of his inventive ways to treat Taylor "outside the box." Taylor had almost completed what seemed to her the impossible, living in Houston for a month. We were both sad to say goodbye to Dr. Anderson but thrilled to go home.

We expected a pleasant last check-in. Taylor was not having any tests, and she felt about as good as you can feel after finishing almost a month of radiation. We smiled when we saw him, ready to bid farewell and thank him for all he had done for Taylor. In his office, Taylor wiggled, crossing and uncrossing her legs, fidgety and eager to get back to the hotel to pack. Her sweet sixteen party was in a few days.

"I'm afraid Taylor may have leukemia," declared Dr. Anderson, avoiding my eyes. In utter confusion, I yelled, "What are you talking about?" His words were, quite frankly, completely out of left field. My brain was screaming. I had feared leukemia, a common side effect of high-dose chemotherapy, but I knew it would never sneak up because Taylor's blood counts were monitored weekly, and no suspicious trends had been noted.

I screeched, "How are you coming to this conclusion?"

He calmly replied that one of Taylor's blood numbers, which I can't currently recall, was consistently high. This was my daughter's life. I believed I understood every blood count number that was significant and not once was the number he was referencing ever mentioned to me as being important. My hysteria grew with each question I asked. His response was consistently vague.

"I need you to call Bob, Dr. Anderson, and explain to him what on earth you are talking about. Because I really don't understand!" Dr. Anderson dialed Bob's office. The call went directly to voicemail. "Hi, Bob, Dr. Anderson here. Please give me a call when you get this message. Thank you." With that, he quietly hung up.

A message? Seriously? I quickly dialed Bob's cell phone and put the phone up to Dr. Anderson's ear. Bob answered and spoke briefly with Dr. Anderson. My heart was racing, desperate for more information, but I couldn't gather much, hearing only one side of the conversation. Bob wasn't buying it, but we needed more than just the views of two very opinionated parents.

I asked, in a voice I did not even recognize as my own, "When will we know for sure?" He replied, "In about two months, around Christmas time." When your child's life is in jeopardy, wondering is not an option. I thought, *I am not waiting until Christmas. There has to be a different way to diagnose leukemia.* Right or wrong, I consistently refused to give the doctors the benefit of the doubt.

Perhaps the craziest part of this frantic experience was that the whole time Dr. Anderson and I were conversing, Taylor was sitting next to me, listening in silence. I literally had a tantrum about her life and possible death while she sat and watched. Clearly, I regret that terribly, but I honestly have no clue what her expression was in that moment.

Taylor indicated to me that she was ready to leave. We walked out the door, and in earshot of Dr. Anderson, Taylor exclaimed, "Fuck him. He is clueless. I don't have leukemia. Let's go to Friday's for baked potato skins." With that, we abruptly left and headed to the infamous Houston mall for lunch, and Taylor didn't worry about it for another minute. Taylor didn't waste much time on worrying.

On October 31, after her six o'clock final radiation treatment, Taylor rang a huge, gold-colored hospital bell indicating her treatment was over. The room applauded. We darted like two birds flying north for the summer to catch our seven-thirty flight home. She vomited on the way out but barely stopped to acknowledge it. At the airport, for the first time, Taylor accepted the medical priorities to which she was entitled. We were picked up at our car with a wheelchair and escorted to the gate. She was Cinderella in her carriage on her way to the ball.

The perfect end to our crazy day awaited us in our driveway at home. As we drove up the street, Taylor saw Bob standing next to a brand-new, baby-blue Volkswagen EOS convertible. "I never thought I would get a car!" she shouted blissfully. "A convertible, Daddy, my favorite color. Thank you sooooooo much! Mommy, look!" She had forgotten that she and Bob had looked at cars while they were in Houston, while he reminisced about the red Volkswagen bug he used to drive. She had pointed out the EOS convertible herself. It was a brand new model and not terribly expensive but it was totally different. It was classic Tales. The joy in her eyes was dwarfed by the love spilling out of Bob's heart. I quickly snapped a picture. Nothing was more satisfying than sending that picture to her doctors with the caption, "This is a life worth living!"

Jordan was there to greet Taylor. They hopped in the car. Bob and I watched as her little baby-blue convertible slowly glided over the cobblestones covering our driveway and whizzed down the street. The smell of a brand-new car, the vision of her hair blowing, the smooth humming of a new engine, and the music blasting filled my senses. Just for a moment, as I watched her zip away, serenity engulfed me. My pulse was rapid, but my mind was calm. The sunshine beat its warm, loving rays upon me, and I could feel, without seeing, the hazy white clouds moving gently across the azure sky. Suddenly it was quiet, the air still and heavy. A deluge of tears burst out: tears of happiness, tears of fear, tears of hope, tears for a future, and tears of joy at how delicious another birthday felt.

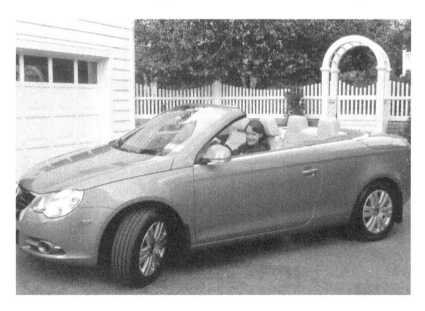

Before we had left Houston, I had contacted Dr. Garvin about Taylor's leukemia scare. Sometimes you need to look for different answers when the ones you're being given don't make any sense. The week we returned home, Dr. Garvin looked at Taylor's blood himself under the microscope and was able to determine immediately that Taylor didn't have leukemia. Again, we had to push the envelope to get a clearer answer. I could have never waited almost two months until Christmas for the results. It truly was a sweet sixteen.

The Sweetest Sixteen

Two luxurious, carpeted, swing-back-chaired coach buses lined up at Edgemont High School to drive the kids into the city. Taylor's sweet sixteen party was at Pacha, a nightclub located on 46th Street in an up-and-coming neighborhood that New Yorkers call Hell's Kitchen.

I repeated to over seventy-five kids, "Excuse me, no gifts allowed on the bus. Our car is parked right there; put them in the trunk." I was met with unfriendly eyes. "Come on, guys. I've known most of you since you were five. You are good kids. Let's not ruin this for Taylor. I know alcohol is stashed in the presents." Those who knew me well laughed, but others were not so pleased. Many sweet sixteen parties had been shut down because of alcohol, and I was taking a big risk bringing underage kids to the city. I didn't want the club to close down the party. Bob and I drove into the city, presents locked in the trunk, while hired chaperones accompanied the kids on the buses, just in case we were tempted to "embarrass" anyone.

When we first began discussing Taylor's sweet sixteen, it was clear she had already done a lot of research. She wanted her party to be at Pacha, a nightclub that held underage parties until midnight, when the club officially opens to the twenty-one-and-over crowd. We went to check it out.

You can imagine my horror, seeing a nightclub during the day. It's like peeling a shiny apple and finding a worm inside. I kept my mouth shut as Taylor and Corey spoke with a fast-talking, attractive young guy who engaged with them quickly. He escorted us to every level of the four-story building. Each floor had its own theme. Taylor picked the level with gray, cushy couches, which must've once been white, flanking a wide-open dance floor with large LED screens on both sides. I knew the deal was sealed upon seeing Taylor's eyes, two huge saucers, and her mouth, slightly agape, almost salivating. I asked, "How did you pick this place?" Tales quickly responded, "This is where I want it to be, *Susssan!*" And so it was. Memories of treatments were already in the rearview mirror. It was time for fun again.

The buses pulled up to Pacha, and the kids came roaring out, ready to party. We snapped away as the kids walked in, catching their smiles and jovial eyes telling us they were ready for a fun night. In groups, they piled into a gray hammered industrial elevator in the lobby.

Taylor looked beautiful, with very little make-up, in a blue satin spaghetti-strapped dress trimmed in black lace and flat silver sandals. The spaghetti straps revealed the many scars along her back, but she never had cared about showing her battle scars. Her nails were painted the exact color of her dress, not an easy task as the blues seen everywhere today were not yet commonplace in nail salons. Taylor's look was completed by a small diamond-and-sapphire necklace, her birthday present from Jordan, which glowed against her pale white skin. Corey's eyes sparkled to match the gold jewelry she was wearing, and her long, lustrous hair was a showstopper. Corey was up for celebrating every moment of her sister's happiness.

Before the party, Jordan had arrived at our house in jeans and a button down. It was obvious he had spent a lot of time on his hair, as it was spiked to perfection. Taylor took one look at him, rolled her eyes, and said, "That shirt looks terrible." Then she blurted out, "You have ten minutes. Get to Andrew's house and borrow that shirt I told you I loved." Taylor said to me, "Isn't he an asshole? I told him what shirt to wear." All I could do was laugh. She was hilarious even when she was being wicked.

Towards the end of the evening Bob got bagels from the iconic H & H bagel shop and dropped a three-foot-high sack on each bus for the ride home. We figured if any of the kids were drunk, bagels would help sober them up. Yes, despite our efforts, we were sure some booze made it in—I remembered too well the time I had filled shampoo bottles with alcohol while away on a school-sponsored trip during my senior year of high school. Some snickered upon seeing the bagels; others burst out laughing, but the sacks were empty when we arrived home.

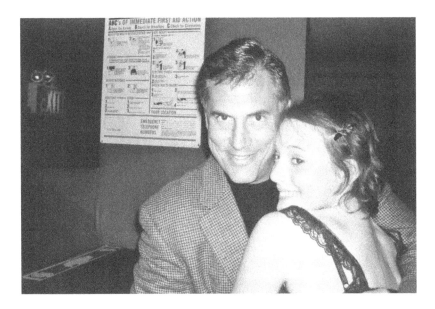

The Will to Persevere

In early December 2007, just over a month after her sweet sixteen party, Taylor walked into the kitchen while I was busy making dinner. Ever so casually, she said, "Mommy, I feel a lump in my neck," yawning while stretching her arms overhead as if it were the first stretch of the day. Showing zero emotion while slowly dying inside, I turned to feel the lump. I told Taylor, "Don't worry; it's a good sign that it moves," but terror swept through me as if someone had a gun to my head. Taylor was fully assuaged by my lack of concern. I called Dr. Carson, who was also our neighbor and whom we affectionately called by her first name, Jessie, and asked for a home visit, knowing full well that house calls were a thing of the past. I was in covert panic mode.

It was twilight on this wintry night in December. I met Jessie at our door with a hot cup of tea and brought her upstairs to my bedroom, where a roaring fire was blazing. My warm room, decorated in tones of blue and green with soft pillows in every corner, was aglow. Taylor sat on a cozy chair snuggled up in a comfy blanket, smiling. Looking in from a distance, it appeared to be a beautiful scene, but one step inside and the tension in the air was palpable. Without showing any emotion, Jessie agreed that it was a good sign that the lump moved, but of course she could not be sure. A CAT scan was scheduled for the next day.

After the scan, Jessie reported with a broad smile and sparkling eyes, "The CAT scan suggested a dark center that might be liquid and, therefore, a classic cyst." We sighed with relief, although we knew we were not quite yet out of the woods—a needle biopsy would tell us for sure. We thought the biopsy would be routine, so Bob went to work as usual, and I took Taylor to the appointment.

The famous Dr. La Quaglia, who had performed the majority of Taylor's surgeries and years later still had a real adoration for her, performed her biopsy at Sloan. He had a pathologist standing by so we could get the biopsy results immediately, understanding I was totally unwilling to wait. Indeed, I had badgered many a doctor for results when they were not forthcoming. Waiting was a form of torture, yet more often than not, results wouldn't be given until days later. I can't grasp why, when a child has cancer, a parent would be made to wait even one unnecessary, excruciating minute for results. Dr. La Quaglia was on our side.

After some Novocain, Tales promptly kicked me out of the surgical room. Taylor, who rarely left my side, was happy to have alone time with Dr. La Quaglia. Apparently, she announced in my absence, "My parents sent me to a butcher for my last surgery. I will never have another surgery with any other doctor than you."

Taylor was famous for speaking her mind from the day she uttered her first word, and this day was no different. When she was little, very early on, she learned the word "no" and never stopped saying it. My father, the jokester, nicknamed Taylor "No."

He would greet her by saying, "Hi, No, do you want candy?"

"NO."

"Taylor, is the sky blue?"

"NO."

It wasn't that she didn't want the candy or know the sky was blue. It was that she couldn't resist being a contrarian.

Moments later, I was conferencing with Dr. La Quaglia. The lump was a cancerous tumor in a lymph node. Full-fledged fear engulfed me, while Tales exuded an ethereal calm. She simply said, "I expected it to be cancer, and I'm ready for surgery."

Dr. La Quaglia looked at us and asked, "When do you want surgery?"

"Tomorrow morning!" we both shouted in unison.

Taylor interjected, with a devilish grin, "I don't like the scar from my last surgery. Can you fix it?"

"I'll do my best. See you tomorrow," he said, winking at Tales.

Giggling, she then added, "I have a date with my boyfriend for dinner and the Radio City Christmas Show tomorrow night. I'm not missing it!"

Dr. La Quaglia, smiling and shaking his head, replied, "Okay, Tales, bring your dress with you."

Getting surgery scheduled for the next day might not sound like much, but many parents wait weeks for Dr. La Quaglia to do his magic. Putting Tales into his surgery schedule at the crack of dawn the next morning made Tales feel rightfully special.

Dr. La Quaglia took out the tumor in short order, found nothing else suspicious in the area, and left the tiny thin scar of a plastic surgeon. Tales soon was back in the recovery room after her *sixteenth* surgery, sore and cranky but able to confirm her date with Jordan. At five in the evening, we left Sloan, and Taylor asked, "Can you and Daddy come along with us tonight?" Imagine, just what Jordan was hoping for—dinner with his girlfriend's parents!

When the bread arrived, Tales stared us down, confirmed she felt fine, and said she was going to the show. When the salad arrived, she was drooping a little but made a fist and insisted on going. When the dessert was offered, she whispered her commitment and fell dead asleep at the table. We put her gently in the car and took her home, Jordan following behind with a sorrowful smile.

Another Christmas by the Sea

Taylor was determined that Jordan, being Jewish, have his first Christmas with us. She went as far as buying him a card and a stocking with the words, in sparkling red and green letters, "Baby's First Christmas." She also invited him to join our family in what was now our new family tradition: Christmas in Sea Island.

It was a true family affair: Aunt Annie and her family flew in from London, my dad from Florida, and my twin brother Paul from New York. My sister Lynn, as usual, didn't join us. She was spending Christmas vacationing in Africa with her family, and sadly, she "didn't have time" even before the holiday to celebrate with us. I was no longer surprised, but I was hurt on behalf of my children.

We arranged for a live Christmas tree in our suite, just like the year before, and on our mantle hung Christmas stockings for all. Everyone's stocking had his or her name embroidered on it, except Jordan's. His "Baby's First Christmas" was left at home and replaced here with one that read, "Santa, I Can Explain."

When Samantha and Sofia arrived, the excitement began rising like steam out of a large cup of cocoa, the aroma of joy filling the air. Taylor had always adored Christmas, and this year she felt she had so much for which to be thankful. She embraced both of her little cousins and raised everyone's exhilaration to an absolute fever pitch.

On Christmas Eve, we went to a tiny and enchanting little chapel nestled in the grounds of the hotel. Covered in ivy, it looked like a church you'd find tucked in the woods somewhere in Austria. We all felt closer to God, and maybe we were. It seemed we had all reached a spiritual level similar to the one Taylor first felt when we took her to midnight mass so many moons before.

Suddenly Jordan jumped up and ran out of the chapel. Taylor looked at me with questioning eyes. I held up my arms indicating, "I have no clue." Apparently, Jordan had to vomit, I guess from a stomach virus. Taylor was pissed, stomach virus or not, and that started the day off on the wrong foot. Patience was not her virtue.

At dinner that night the tables were set with lustrous ivory linens and adorned with glowing candles, creating an atmosphere of elegance and beauty. Everyone was dressed up and ready for a glorious evening when Jordan, again, bolted, with great urgency, from the table. Taylor's expression fit her words, "What the hell?" as she ran after him, only to find him vomiting once again.

He didn't return for quite a while. She thought he was overreacting. Despite all the times he comforted her while she was ill, she was having none of it. "Are you kidding me, Jordan? I vomited for years from chemo, and you have a stupid bug and are ruining Christmas Eve for me. Go home!" Jordan, weak, pale, and exhausted, didn't say a word. Later Taylor relayed to me, with anger and disappointment, "Jordan's mom changed his flight. He's leaving tomorrow," followed by, "I am *not* sleeping in an adjoining room to him. Can I sleep on your couch, Mommy?"

Before the little kids went to bed, Taylor gave them, and everyone else, matching cherry-red flannel Christmas pajamas covered in snowmen and snowflakes. She had purchased them just before we headed to Sea Island. Everyone donned their outfits, and the girls helped Samantha write a note to Santa. She left him yummy cookies and a precious note, but the real fun began when Uncle Bill got involved. As he does every year, he left Santa a few gifts of his own, including rotten onions, an old sock, and fart "candy." Uncle Bill's note told Santa, aka "The Pant Load," to stay off his roof and go on a diet, among other things. It set the tone for good fun and a lot of laughs, but Taylor was crestfallen.

As soon as I awoke the next morning, I looked from our bed to see Taylor snuggled up on the couch. Her face was peaceful and calm, shining from the soft glow of the Christmas tree lights. Just watching the rise and fall of her breath filled my heart with pure happiness. I wondered if anything had transpired while I was asleep.

I found out later that morning that, by text message, the two lovebirds had indeed reconciled overnight. Jordan appeared the next morning, pale and embarrassed, but shortly thereafter his bad mood and his virus faded away. Months or maybe years later, I looked at my credit card bills for a reason I cannot recall, and I saw a charge of seventy-five dollars posted on that Christmas morning. She got me again! If she were here, she would be laughing, saying, "Mommy, we had to pay the change fee on Jordan's flight so he didn't have to go home." Not surprisingly, Taylor had memorized my credit card number.

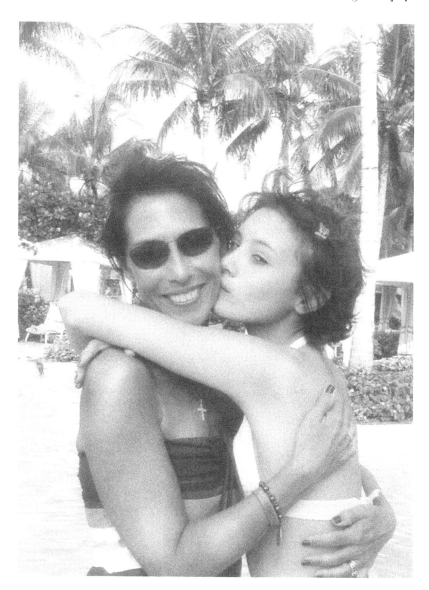

Little Miss Bo Peep

With New Year's 2008 approaching, Taylor asked me without missing a beat, "What medications shouldn't I take so I can drink on New Year's?" I responded simply, "I don't know. You need to ask." I knew that New Year's Eve meant more drinking than normal. So Taylor asked Jane, our nurse practitioner, who was very cautious. In a serious tone, she answered, "Sue,

Taylor is underage! How can you allow her to drink?" In all fairness to Jane, she doesn't have children, but I thought to myself, *How unrealistic can you be?* Taylor and I both tried not to burst out laughing, but we couldn't contain ourselves. Jane was always extremely kindhearted and, in true Jane form, wasn't offended. She simply looked at us and matter-of-factly stated, "Okay, let's ask Dr. Garvin."

Taylor entered the examining room wearing her signature smirk and blurted out, "Dr. Garvin, is it okay for me to drink, and what meds can't I take?" Without raising his head from her chart, he replied, "Just don't take any of the narcotics you're using for your back pain." Jane was silent as red splotches crept up her face, and she soon could not conceal her blush. Of course, that made Tales laugh even harder. The New Year was beginning on a happy note, but as always, I wondered what a new year would bring.

Months later, I relayed that story to Taylor's friend Jessie, who was always up for fun. She burst out into laughter just as Taylor had. I was puzzled. How could the joke now be on me?

"Sue, really? Taylor had been drinking all along. You should've seen her on Halloween, dressed up like Little Bo Peep! She was definitely wasted."

"But she had been taking so many meds, how did she know if it was safe?"

All Jessie could say was, "Well, nothing happened."

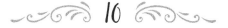

10

Going Rogue

I literally have to remind myself all the time, that being afraid of things going wrong isn't the way to make things go right.

–dau-@cosmicextension

The Beginning of the End

Midway through January, my sweetheart Corey and I spent the weekend at Canyon Ranch, a spa and wellness center in Massachusetts. She had been starved of "mommy time" for almost five years, and we needed some time alone. While there, Bob called and reported, "I took Taylor and Jordan to their favorite place, Dave & Busters, and she drove!" With only a permit, I was shocked that Taylor had driven over the Tappan Zee, a large, six-lane bridge. But she showed no fear.

"And I took them to a steak dinner at Ruth's Chris." Then Bob added in a low voice, "Taylor had a lot of trouble walking across the parking lot. She had to stop for a break and barely made it up the stairs." This was uncharacteristic of Taylor. No matter what, she always forged ahead. "Oh, no," I sobbed. Bob insisted I stay at Canyon Ranch, telling me, "I will watch her." I knew he would take every precaution, and I was happy they were having a great weekend together, but sirens were sounding in my head.

Corey and I were getting manicures the next day when the phone rang again. I recognized the number as one of Taylor's oncologists. No cell phones were allowed in the spa, but I picked up regardless. "Hello?" I whispered. "Hi, Sue. I just saw Bob and Taylor at the hospital. They are en route home, but I want her to come back for a chest x-ray." In a total panic, I dialed Bob. "Bob, they want you to return to the hospital for an x-ray." On speakerphone, Taylor sternly replied, "No, I'm going home to see Jordan." She was mad as hell about having to return to the hospital. All I know is, on our end, in a matter of moments, Corey packed up our entire room and we frantically checked out.

The weather in Lenox, Massachusetts, was bone chilling. I stopped for gas, totally annoyed at the five additional minutes it would cost me. While I was filling up, Bob called and said, "Taylor's chest x-ray was okay." What? Shocked, I took a breath and decided to go into the convenience store to buy lottery tickets, just as we always used to do on road trips. This was the closest Corey had come to normalcy in a long time.

When we arrived home, I was stunned when I saw Taylor. I had only been away for three days. What had happened? Taylor's cancer had suddenly gone rogue. She was beginning to struggle for every breath. I was scared—the kind of scared that, as humans, we're unable to fully imagine until we experience it. Shaking from the inside out, I remember being unable to easily breathe myself. Taylor had visibly deteriorated in just a few days.

Giving up hope was not an option. We made plans to go to Germany in a few weeks for a protocol Bob had been investigating and arranging for more than two years, in case Taylor relapsed and treatments available in the United States weren't working. Back when Bob was first investigating, Tales had asked her favorite history teacher, Ms. Pearlman, a petite blonde who loved helping her students, to show her maps from modern Germany after they became a unified nation. She explained, "If I relapse, Daddy has a plan to take me to Germany for treatment." Together they examined the map for quite a while, as if Taylor was searching for clues to plan her itinerary for a wondrous trip. She was always one step ahead, right along with Bob.

The treatment was predicated on using one's own immune system to naturally attack and hopefully eradicate the cancer, and the procedure mandated taking Taylor's tumor cells, mixing them with her own "natural killer cells" and dendritic cells in a petri dish, and adding a virus to trigger an immune response whereby her own cells would multiply into the millions. The resulting "natural killer cells" and dendritic cells were to be injected back into her bloodstream. The hope was that this process would awaken Taylor's immune system and her body would recognize her cancer as foreign and eviscerate it. I had to believe that this would work.

Before we headed to Germany, Taylor was scheduled to take the New York State Regents exams. I pleaded, "Taylor, this is ridiculous; the exams will be given again in June." She told me, in no uncertain terms, "Mommy, I am taking them because they are required to graduate in New York State. Sorry, but end of story."

I didn't want to argue with her about this, but it was incredibly obvious that she needed oxygen. I dropped her off at school and called the hospital in search of in-home oxygen tanks. Jane matter-of-factly responded, "Really? Why do you need them? We saw Taylor last week and she was fine. Bring her in after school, and we will evaluate her." I replied, "Fine, but order the tanks now!"

Now that she was older, on the days Taylor went to school, she had a habit of not coming home at the end of the day but instead gallivanting off with her friends or Jordan. I called her teacher at school and told her, "Make sure Taylor meets me in the back parking lot after school so I can take her to the hospital." It was uncharacteristic of a parent to call about their eleventh grader, and I could feel just the tiniest bit of surprise from her teacher. I bellowed, "Taylor cannot breathe. She is faking it, and I need her!" I cannot imagine what her teacher thought.

Jordan brought Taylor to the car and came with us to the hospital. Jane asked, "Taylor, can you take a lap around the hospital floor?" Taylor responded, "No, I can't without oxygen." My eyes met Jane's. Panic set it.

It suddenly dawned on me that Taylor was faking her ability to breathe not only with her friends, teachers, and nurses, but with us as well. I asked her, "Why?" I remember her response vividly, and I can still recall the sound of her voice. She calmly stated, "I don't want to be like Nana," referring to my mother. "Nana freaked out when she couldn't breathe and took so many anti-anxiety drugs, like you. Mommy, I just stay calm and figure out ways to catch my breath."

Taylor agreed, on her terms, to use oxygen during the second part of the Regents. "Mommy, *pleeeease* arrange it so they can hide me from the other students. I don't want anyone to see me with an oxygen tank."

On Taylor's last day of the Regents Exam, she was scheduled to have scans, which meant she could not eat all day. I begged, "Taylor, stay home and sleep. Don't take the Regents on an empty stomach," to which she emphatically replied, "NO." Over the years, we had tried desperately to spare Taylor from suffering. Morning scans helped. But these were emergency scans, and we had to take what we could get.

In the waiting area, she asked, "Mommy, can I have pain medication? My back is killing me." I immediately gave it to her, but by now I should have known better. *Damn it, Sue!* It hadn't dawned on me that I was giving Taylor a narcotic on an empty stomach. The effects were devastating. Taylor had to lay still in a CT/PET scan for over an hour. When the scan was over, she tried to sit up and immediately vomited uncontrollably. Her frail little body had nothing left. It took forty-five minutes to get her off the table to a chair and another hour to get her out of the radiologist's office.

With difficulty, she walked to the car and was silent the entire ride home. I didn't know if she had remembered that her friend Sarah, who was leaving the next day for a semester abroad, was coming over to visit. As I settled her in bed, she casually asked, "Is Sarah coming?" I replied, "Only if you want her to." She looked at me like I was crazy. "Duh, of course I want to see her." I smiled. She was on to the next source of fun. Never, ever count Taylor out.

Love Is All You Need

My hands shook as I picked up the phone to call Andrea, who was living in London. "Andrea," my voice a mere whisper in between sobs, "it's time to come home. *Taylor can't breathe anymore.*"

The screams and sobs on both ends of the phone made it impossible for us to speak or hear each other. After a few minutes, Andrea asked, "Is Ryan coming home?"

"Yes, I told her to come, but I haven't told her how bad it is yet. I just can't bear to scare her, and I don't think Tales thinks it's as bad as it is."

Then, in a complete turnaround, Andrea reminded me, "You know, Tales always pulls through. She will this time, too; you'll see. She's been in worse situations before and made it." I had to agree. She seemed to go way past the nine lives of a cat. She had as many as she needed.

I called my dad in Florida. I don't recall my conversation with him, but I imagine I used the same words: "It's time to come." He arrived the next morning.

Andrea, Bill, and Samantha arrived a day later to a very frail Taylor, still walking but on oxygen 100 percent of the time. Andrea's in-laws had graciously hopped on a flight from Boston to London to babysit one-year-old Sofia, but their flights crossed in the air, so Andrea had left Sofia with a babysitter until they arrived, not knowing if her in-laws were arriving on time and not being able to communicate with them. Anything for Taylor.

I asked Taylor if she would like a visit from Aunt Lynn. For years, Taylor would say, "Mommy, you're being too harsh. Give Aunt Lynn the benefit of the doubt." For a while, I wondered if my anger about Taylor's situation had tainted my judgment. But when I asked Taylor who she wanted to visit her, she did not include Aunt Lynn or her daughters. When I asked why, she answered very matter-of-factly, "Mommy, they obviously don't love me. Why would I want to see them now?" There it was, and it confirmed that I hadn't misunderstood Lynn's actions. Taylor, who was always unbiased and tried to see the best in her aunt, had finally admitted to herself the cold, hard truth.

My brother, who lived fifteen minutes away, arrived, too. His eyes and tone betrayed his fear; he looked at Taylor like she was dying. I pulled him into another room, shut the door, and explained, "You are not allowed to see Taylor with that look on your face; get it together if you want to enjoy any time with her." He replied, "Aren't you going to invite Lynn and her girls over, too? You really should."

My daughter was on death's door, and he had the nerve to talk about Lynn. I was furious. I screamed, "Why should they come? Taylor hasn't seen them in months and doesn't want to see them. Her girls declined an invitation to Taylor's sweet sixteen, and then Lynn cancelled plans with us for Christmas. If Taylor saw them now, out of the blue, she would know something was wrong. Sorry, but there is no way I can risk her knowing that this may be the end. She's still *fighting*. I need to protect her."

Naturally, Tales had asked, "Why are you guys here, Aunt Annie?" Andrea came up with a suitable answer, as the floor below her seemed to buckle. We certainly couldn't tell Taylor the real reason. Andrea said, "You know, Tales, we're repatriating from London, so we came to look at houses in Connecticut. Soon, I'm going to live close by. You're going to see me so much you're going to get so sick of seeing me." Taylor smiled wide, eyes aglow like she had just been given the gift of a lifetime, and shook her head. "Never."

Later in the week, Taylor seemed to be breathing easier, and we began thinking that her shortness of breath was perhaps a symptom of infection instead of a growing tumor. Our spirits rose. Was she making yet another comeback? Taylor wanted to take the whole family to a popular restaurant, X2O, run by the famous Chef Peter Kelly and where Jordan was interning. We got dressed up, and just before we were about to leave, we asked Samantha to go upstairs and see if Taylor was ready so Bob could carry her down. He had been carrying Taylor up and down the steps for the past few weeks because she couldn't make the stairs on her own. As we waited for Taylor's reply, she shocked us all by walking down the steps, hand in hand with Samantha—smile wide, fierce determination in her eyes, *without* her oxygen tank.

Just a week earlier, she couldn't take a lap around the hospital clinic without oxygen, and she hadn't been without it since. I whispered to Bob, "Is she really planning on going to dinner without oxygen?" I didn't really have to ask because I already knew the answer. She was jubilant and defiant and enjoying our reaction. Again, our fears of losing her were subsiding. So many times over the years, we could have lost Taylor, but she always managed to pull through.

Taylor often said, "When Aunt Annie comes, I always get better." Well, Aunt Annie's magic had worked again. No one could believe her grit, and to this day, I believe it was the love shared during that week that strengthened her. Taylor's cancer had invaded her body, torn it apart, and left her with half her lung capacity, a body crisscrossed with scars, and horrible back pain. Yet as she walked down those steps, I could still see the little girl with boundless energy who used to run laps around our house with a big smile and bright-red cheeks.

During that time, Taylor was basically confined to her bedroom, a place she loved, and her large oxygen tank was stationed there. She spent a good part of the day playing the Wii, an electronic interactive video game that was all the rage in 2008, with Uncle Billy Boy. Their favorite game was tennis. Watching them "whack" the digital balls over the net as if they were actually dueling on a clay court was a sight to be seen. Bill would jump up, whacking the air with a loud grunt, and Taylor would whack the ball back, playing in bed, laughing.

Ryan returned home from college that Friday night. Now we were really ready to have some fun! Together our two families always laughed until our bellies hurt, even in the most harrowing of circumstances. Being all together made us feel high, as if someone had spiked our drinks, and laughing until the tears streamed out was commonplace. But it was out of character, even for us, when Andrea and I decided to perform and sing the music to *The Rocky Horror Picture Show*. Of course, we knew the entire accompanying dance moves as well. The kids thought we had lost our minds. They had never heard of *Rocky Horror*, let alone the song, "Let's Do the Time Warp Again." They busted out with laughter, and somehow, we were able to purely have fun in the moment.

On Sunday, Ryan gathered everything she needed for the ultimate Super Bowl party. It was particularly important because the New York Giants, our home team, were playing the New England Patriots, Uncle Bill's home team who had just completed a perfect season. My dad is the ultimate Giants fan, having held season tickets for over thirty years.

"Mom, I'm going to Modell's to pick up red shirts for the Patriots and blue shirts for the Giants and iron-on decals!" exclaimed Ryan.

"No one's rooting for the Patriots except Bill," declared Andrea.

"Not so fast, Aunt Annie," replied Tales, "Daddy and I are Eagles fans so we are rooting for New England!"

"What? You guys live in New York! You can't be serious." But they were. Taylor could never resist teaming up with Uncle Billy Boy.

Next came the food. "I got red and blue jellybeans, and red and blue icing for the cake," said Ryan, the ultimate party planner. "Okay, Tales, here's the deal," chided Aunt Annie. "Put all the red and blue jellybeans in a bowl, mix them up, and then close your eyes and pick a handful. If you pick more blue, the Giants will win, and if you pick more red, the Patriots will win." There were about two hundred jellybeans in the bowl. Taylor scooped up a big handful, and everyone watched to see which team would prove victorious.

"Oh my gosh! I don't believe it!" We were stunned as Taylor had picked an entire handful of *only blue* jellybeans!

"The Giants are going to win. Ha, ha!" exclaimed Andrea. Of course, no one really believed that. The Giants were massive underdogs. But as great as the odds were against the Giants, even greater were the odds of blindly picking, out of two hundred mixed jellybeans, all one color—her favorite color.

We gathered around our big-screen TV in our varying red and blue team T-shirts. Taylor startled me once again by taking off her oxygen. We huddled together, enjoying the game, but more important, we marveled at how well Tales was doing and how she was completely immersed in the festivities, having seemingly forgotten about her troubles.

The game was particularly riveting, given that it was closer than expected, and Andrea, Paul, and my dad, true Giants fans, were going nuts, hoping for the impossible. And then it happened, just as Taylor "predicted." In the fourth quarter, down 14–10, the Giants got the ball on their own seventeen-yard line and, with only two minutes left, scored the winning touchdown. We chalked it up to one of those psychic "coincidences" that seemed to always come up when Taylor was around.

The next morning, Ryan and Taylor embraced to say goodbye. As always, they were sad to separate. When my dad left, Taylor said, "Feel well, Pop-Pop," to which he responded, "Taylor, you feel well, too," believing it might be their last exchange. Mercifully, I was not present, because I think I would have lost it. My mother had passed away ten months earlier, and Taylor worried constantly about Pop-Pop. "Mommy, do you think he will die, too? You know that sometimes happens." I reassured her that he was fine, but in those ten months, Taylor repeated the question many times. And yet, as I write this, Pop-Pop just celebrated his eighty-sixth birthday and is in good health.

Andrea closed her suitcase to return to London, looking at the dark suit she had packed—just in case it really was the end. She had done the same when she visited our mother last year and ended up staying for her funeral. She thought, *Taylor, if you only knew that I packed for your funeral.* It made her weep but then smile, because, of course, Taylor ended up defying the odds.

The next day, when Andrea, Bill, and Samantha left, Corey and Taylor were somber but otherwise clueless. Young, adorable Samantha, with her wispy blonde hair and tiny frame, smiled at Taylor devilishly. She was as mischievous as her role model. "Play your violin for me, Sammie," requested Tales, smiling. Samantha proudly obliged and played us a melody, the notes of which seemed only for us, gracing Taylor with her love for the last time.

Brown, a University Built on Distinction

Brown University was Taylor's first choice. She wanted to visit, fully believing she might attend one day, so we went with it, no hesitation.

Exhausted from our week of visitors, we were quiet in the car ride up, and when we checked into our hotel, we immediately got into bed. Next to my bed was a Bible. It was the first time I had ever reached for the Bible to look for answers and hope. I opened to a random page and was astounded to find words of comfort. Just like that, my faith in a good outcome returned. I felt God was sending me a sign.

The next day, as we entered the campus entrance, we passed the beautifully ornate, massive, and impressive Van Winkle Gates, which displayed the Brown University shield. "This is where you will enter at commencement and where you will exit at convocation," said the tour guide. Apparently, the main gate is closed except for these momentous times of the year. Taylor smiled at me with "that look," which I interpreted to mean, "I got it, Mom. I am walking in and out." She looked so happy, so proud of all of her achievements. I felt keenly the paradox of this moment: the fixed symbol marking the beginning and end of the university journey, and my own mind bouncing like a ball between my joy at her elation and my horror at what might be her reality.

As we continued around campus, I glanced over at Taylor, who was clearly struggling for breath, far too proud to use her oxygen on the university tour. Yet she soaked up every word the tour guide spoke, her questions abounding. When we passed a dorm with treadmills, Taylor pointed and said, "See, now I can do my pulmonary rehabilitation here rather than at that gloomy and pathetic rehab center." Really, Tales? Treadmills? She always focused on the future.

When we entered the admissions building for the information session, Taylor looked at the stairs with trepidation. After all the kids had reached the top, without a word, Bob scooped Taylor up in his arms and carried her upstairs. She looked back at me with a huge grin.

As we were listening to the admissions presentation, Taylor began falling asleep due to the exertion of the campus tour and her low levels of oxygen. I insisted, "Taylor, I have a portable tank right here in my bag; no one will notice the tubing. You don't have a choice!" She gave in and perked up as the oxygen filled her compromised lungs. When the session ended, she approached the front of the room to speak with a thin, graying man who stood tall, clearly very proud of the university, and inquired about the curriculum. She was overjoyed with his confirmation that she could construct her own major. As we walked away, she asked, "Where is the closest hospital? Mommy, I'm so sorry I won't be eighteen until November of my freshman year. I know you'll have to travel here every week so I can get my treatment for the first few months." Before I could respond, she added rather flippantly, "I can take care of it myself after that."

A few days later, Taylor was scheduled to have a surgical procedure at Sloan to blast, by radio frequency ablation, some of the more threatening nodules in her lungs. Yet she refused to go to pre-op, telling me, "Mommy, I won't miss my first driver's ed class!"

Prior to the procedure, Bob spoke with the radiologists to determine the most effective way to get at the bigger cancerous tumors, to give Taylor more breathing capacity. I don't know why Bob was shocked to see that the radiologist did not have the most recent scan; we had encountered so many medical errors.

Luckily Bob had the most recent scan on his laptop, and the doctor used that to proceed.

With radio frequency ablation, the idea is to not only damage the cancerous tumors but also possibly set off an immune response. Taylor and Bob had both read all of the research. After surgery, the radiologist came to see us, advising that the procedure did not go well and Taylor was bleeding too much. As we continued to ask questions, his body language revealed his concerns. We continued to ask, "When she was scoped, what did you see?" He was clearly spooked, and we knew it. He was backpedaling out of the room ever so slowly so he could escape as quickly as possible. In the elevator taking Taylor to recovery, we asked his fellow, "Why did Taylor bleed so much?" He very matter-of-factly said, "That is totally normal; it happens all the time." *So why did they abort?*

The next day, Taylor had one of her typical inpatient days, laughing with her visiting friends. My treasured friends Lori and Jeanne arrived, and Jeanne told me later, "I had a lengthy discussion with Tales. She told me that she wanted to grow up just like you and have friends for twenty-five or more years." She told Jeanne, "Long and loving friendships are what life's about." That's just what she was hoping for.

The Perfect Storm

Later that week, Taylor was due for chemo, and we had an appointment to see her oncology consultant Dr. Chang, a husky Asian man with a huge presence and a permanently serious and straightforward demeanor. We had been consulting with him for years. His practice combined Eastern and Western medicine, but more important, he was known for telling the truth about treatments and combinations of drugs not approved in the United States but available overseas. He had suggested the treatment in Germany years ago, but we had been too scared to take Tales off chemo to try it. Now we were going to get our final instructions for our trip. My friend Barbara was staying with Taylor in clinic until I could get the car and pick them up. Barbara had spent so many horrifying days with us in the hospital. She ran as fast as I did whenever Taylor wanted something.

I exited the elevator at Columbia and was distraught to see a major snowstorm developing. In a matter of minutes, snow blanketed the streets, each flake so large you could almost make out its individual intricacies. Unbeknownst to us, a blizzard had been forecasted. As I departed the building, handing in my valet ticket, a tumultuous gust of wind pierced through me, assaulting my personal space and quickly pervading my thoughts.

Dr. Chang's office was located downtown, completely across town from Columbia, which could mean at least an hour in traffic under normal conditions. Hot tears rolled down my face faster than the snowflakes. The car wasn't coming up from the hospital valet. Frantically waving my car ticket, I looked for my favorite valet, whose mane of bright-red hair could never be missed, and screamed above the roar of the wind, "I'm going to get the car myself!" Without gloves, a hat, or boots, I ran downhill toward the parking garage. The landscape looked like crystal as the light bounced off the white snowflakes, a beautiful scene to those looking out their windows but not to those who were driving. With adrenaline pumping and chills permeating my body, I began to panic.

I couldn't help but remember that Taylor was born right around the time of the "Perfect Storm," the storm that inspired the movie of the same name. The Perfect Storm was a result of three large weather systems colliding, causing a calamitous trilogy of "apocalyptic trepidation." Apparently this set of weather circumstances occurs approximately every fifty to one hundred years. From the moment Taylor's little hands and feet hit the floor, she had the drive to conquer, persevere, and accelerate everything in her life. I called her "the perfect storm baby," and she loved it!

Now we were facing a storm of our own. I was driving a silver, eight-passenger SUV that stood so high off the ground it took two hands to get into, and its height had always helped when driving through snow. However, the driving conditions were becoming more treacherous by the minute. Next to me, Taylor looked calm but didn't say a word, nor did Barbara, who remained still, if not wide-eyed, in the back seat.

As I looked out my window, it was as if a fairy had cast a spell and frozen the world in time. Although I was desperate to get to our appointment, I could not help but admire the beauty of the soft snow drifting and how artistically the snow was falling. The storm was a dramatic juxtaposition of beauty and serenity, destruction and sorrow. Had Mother Nature meant to be evil and powerful, or soft and beautiful? Or, perhaps, most likely, a little bit of both? As you'll recall, that was a question Taylor often pondered.

Just then I received a call from FedEx. "Mrs. Matthews, we have a package addressed to you that says 'danger, live cells, bio hazardous.'" I knew the package contained a section of Taylor's tumor that we had frozen and housed in a very specific way after her surgery in January 2007. It was essential that we bring it to Germany for her treatment. "We cannot release it from our FedEx office in Memphis." For obvious reasons, I understood why FedEx would stop shipment. I didn't know what to do; I couldn't think. I was terrified to drive while my thoughts were drifting to the impending threat that we wouldn't receive Taylor's tumor cells in time to take them to Germany.

My mind was racing with questions. The institution sending the tumor cells sent samples all over the world. This was routine for them. Why did they package the box that way? How did it make it from where it originated in California to Memphis, where FedEx stopped it? And how the hell was I going to convince FedEx to send it to me?

I had maybe an hour to get the box out of Memphis to have a shot at getting it to New York in time for our departure to Germany. It was a race I was not going to lose. Hell hath no fury like a mother trying to save her child.

I quickly called our dear friend Tom, whose imposing height, piercing blue eyes, bald head, and feisty disposition made him seem larger than life. Once again, this lifesaving connection was courtesy of my friend, Donna, who was dating him at the time. Tom was a private investigator and former deputy chief of police for the NYPD, and I knew he had many connections.

"Tom, Taylor's tumor is stuck in FedEx in Memphis. Can you help?" I shrieked.

"Sue, what are you talking about?"

Against the odds and with a won't-take-no-for-an-answer attitude, Tom was able to run interference and get the box through. I never asked how he did it.

Through it all, Taylor remained uncharacteristically silent. Her fingers turned white as she grasped the seat with what looked like spine-tingling, heart-stopping fear. Her body was rigid; she was losing the little color she had in her face, and her eyes betrayed her severe panic. Although she had overheard the FedEx conversation, it was the severe weather that was really bothering her.

We finally arrived at Dr. Chang's office. Taylor began wiggling in her chair. She asked, "Where's the bathroom?" Dr. Chang pointed without raising his head. The bathroom was down an elongated, almost vertical staircase of probably thirty steps. I can't recall if she had her oxygen with her or not, but I do recall that, as we walked down the steps together, I had no idea how she was going to make it back up. When she came out of the bathroom, she told me, point blank, "I refuse to walk up slowly!" Then she whispered, "Here I go." She took the challenge with the expression of a seasoned marathon runner.

She arrived at the top, desperately gasping for air. She could not speak but motioned to me to hide her in a corner of the waiting room for fear Dr. Chang would see how sick she really was. She was afraid he wouldn't support the trip to Germany. Breathing seemed to be impossible. Yet Taylor did not panic, but simply stood in the corner until she regained her composure.

As she worked on catching her breath, I don't think she noticed my quivering hands, the terror in my face, or the cold sweat sliding down my body. I desperately wanted to breathe for her. I frantically looked through my bag for my anti-anxiety medications—for me, not her. When Taylor's breath normalized, she walked into Dr. Chang's office as if nothing had happened. We received our treatment plans for our trip to Germany and left almost immediately.

Darkness had fallen, and the storm was more tumultuous than ever. Gusts of wind were thrashing around us at a fever pitch. Taylor swiftly covered her mouth with her scarf and somehow got to the car. By then the city was veiled in almost fifteen inches of snow. The only way I could drive was to follow the taillights of the few other cars in front of us. My windshield wipers were covered with heavy ice as they swished back and forth. Visibility had diminished to less than a few yards. Taylor begged me to get off the road, screaming, "MOMMY! We are going to die! We're going to die!" still worried only about the storm.

A Perfect Valentine

Valentine's Day 2008 proved to be a whirlwind of excitement and future plans. Taylor's SAT scores were due to post any moment. All night Tales checked to see if her scores had arrived, with me dozing alongside her in her bed. Ryan had never been as anxious to get her scores and certainty didn't stay up all night. Her scores finally posted around five in the morning. With joy she exclaimed, "Mommy, wake up Daddy!" to which I responded, "Of course, I'm running!" My mind was ablaze with happiness amidst a stabbing sadness that she couldn't sprint for joy to wake her daddy up herself like a normal teen would, as she was tied to an oxygen tank. Bob, hair rustled with sleep, sprinted into her room. Taylor beamed and said, "I think I can go to Brown University now!"

Taylor's topnotch SAT scores did not surprise us, although they should have, considering that she missed more school than she attended and was constantly compromised by treatment and surgery. On the day that Taylor took the test, she could barely walk. She was tethered to an oxygen machine with the level turned way up. And still she was blue.

Later that day, Tales asked, "Can you drop me off at Jordan's so we can celebrate Valentine's Day?" After a short time, Jordan called me in a panic: "Tales' oxygen tank ran out!" I was calm, as I knew Taylor would be. I instructed him, "Carry her to the car, and I will be waiting in our driveway with a new tank." T was not unsettled at all but Jordan was clearly spooked.

Only after we lost her did I find the letter she wrote to Jordan that Valentine's Day on her computer:

Dear Jordan,

Today is Valentine's Day, and I sat down to write you a card, but I just keep feeling like something is wrong. See, I'm asking myself, what is Valentine's Day? February 14, is that all? Today is a day when love is supposedly in the air, and everyone buys flowers and chocolate, wears red and pink, and tries to be romantic. But, Jordan, you do not need a holiday to do this. Every day of my life, I wake up so happy to be in love with such a caring and amazing person. Every day you are romantic. You tell me you love me, and you make me feel love in the air when no one else can see it.

This past year has been incredible. We have grown so close so fast; you have been there for me through everything and continue to be always. Of course, we have our fights and our rough times, but we always manage to kiss and make up (even if sometimes that is more than a kiss). You have successfully put up with, and hopefully learned to love, one of the most difficult and stubborn people in the world (aka me). In order to do this, you must be a spectacular person. You have won the hearts of my entire family who now care about you as if you were a part of the family, and you have supported each one of us in our turn, whether you recognize it or not. By far, you are the most considerate boyfriend ever, and I know that you would do anything you could to make me happy, as would I for you.

Jordan, even more than I want you to know how much I love you loving me, I want you to know how much I love you. Every day with you is a blessing. I wake up thanking God that I have you and wondering where I would be without you. I love being there for you, helping you, and watching you prove to people that you are worth more than they think you are because, Jordan, you are worth much more than most people I know. The fact that I found you and you found me when we were just in high school just adds to the romanticism of this unfolding love tale that extends into our future. Jordan, I cannot imagine a life without you, and I never want to find out how I would have to live it. We will never be in an open relationship—I know you have been worrying about that—because I want you, Jordan, and only you, always and forever,

I LOVE YOU. Happy Valentine's Day!

Love, Taylor

Valentine's Day was filled with future dreams of growing up, going to college, and loving Jordan.

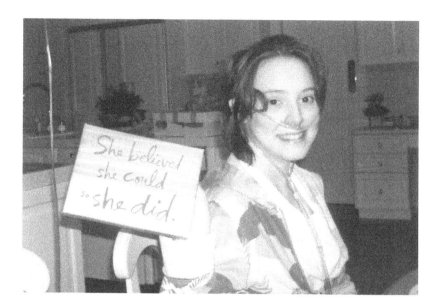

Everything's Okay If
I'm with Tay

*The risk of love is loss and the price of loss is grief. But the pain of
grief is only a shadow compared with the pain of never risking love.*

–Hillary Stanton Zunin

Terror in the Air

Although Taylor was in abysmal shape, had been tethered to an oxygen
tank for three weeks, and was having difficulty walking, it was time to
go to Germany. I bargained with God once again, praying for a cure
in Germany. I promised I would do anything to help others, take on the cancer
myself, or go blind, an odd fear I still carry.

In preparation for the trip, I arranged for enough oxygen to travel to the
airport in New York, our nine-hour flight, and for oxygen to be delivered to our
hotel in Germany. It was no easy feat. I put out a call for help. Within minutes,
my petite, spunky, and spontaneous friend Lori left her desk in New Jersey and

drove straight to our home. Taylor embraced her with a huge smile and quickly asked, "Can I have a foot massage?" Taylor was crazy for Lori's foot massages. I gave them any old cream I could put my hands on and left. I heard the two of them bursting in laughter as they realized the cream had glitter in it. I glanced into the room and saw my bedcover filled with glitter. Happiness filled my heart.

Another dear friend, Donna, ran in and out. I have never asked her to know for sure, but I sensed she knew it was going to be the last time she would see Taylor, and I imagine she just couldn't bear it.

Taylor's friends and Jordan came during their lunch periods to visit her, so she was entertained all day.

Later Janet, my dear friend who had spontaneously invited Ryan to Rome last year, arrived, and she and Taylor chatted as they had for years. Janet, with her warm and nurturing heart, now says, with tears in her eyes, "I was so thrilled to have her to myself." An exclusive one-on-one with T was rare. Janet eventually said her goodbyes when Diana arrived.

Diana, Bob's executive assistant, was like a member of the family. Diana has a presence about her. It isn't just her thick, luxurious black hair that cascades down her back or her tall stature and confident air; it's the kindness that emanates from within, the slight wrinkles that betray her smiling eyes.

Diana knew the whole story from the beginning and she understood that if this trip was going to happen, it was going to need organization, logistics, and clear thinking. Diana presented Taylor with what she called "The Book," which not only outlined our flights and hotels in Germany but also served as a scrapbook overflowing with pictures and historical notes about everywhere we were going, including Vienna. We were planning on incubating Taylor's cells once we got overseas, and in the four days it would take to cultivate them, we were going to meet Andrea and her family in Vienna for a vacation. The doctors advised us otherwise, but as usual, we refused to be scared into submission.

Diana realized we were over our heads but was trying to be subtle. She had offered to come with us on a last-minute basis, but Bob had said no. He was worried that she didn't understand what she was getting into. Suddenly, Taylor pulled me aside and whispered, "Can Diana come on the trip?" I responded, "Maybe. But you have to ask Daddy." Taylor was nervous about asking, but of course, Bob agreed. Taylor was right. We needed Diana. And she needed clothes, a passport, and a ticket, which she quickly arranged.

Now, we were set. We were a team, setting out for a cure and a week in Europe—except Ryan, who remained at Wake Forest. I had convinced myself this trip was not the end, so I saw no reason to take her out of school. Again, my on-again, off-again reality told me Taylor would be fine.

The next morning Taylor's friends Jenny and Laura came over with Starbucks and other goodies. I poked my head into her room and saw them on her bed, laughing and chatting like normal teenagers. After Taylor left her room that day for the final time, I stared at it and thought, *Could this be the last time she ever sees her beloved room?* I quickly dismissed that idea, thinking, *At least she'll never see it looking like it does, in complete disarray*, because I knew her room would be cleaned while we were away. I am still dumbfounded that I was able to rationalize everything.

Just before we departed for the airport, right on cue, Barbara and her son Sandy arrived to say good-bye. He and Tales laughed, played a game, and carried on with their usual banter. I believe Barbara knew it might be the last time she saw Taylor—her shining blue eyes were dull and her face a bit ashen—but Sandy said goodbye in his usual sweet manner.

We arrived at JFK to a mysteriously empty terminal with no airline attached to it. Two airline agents stood military style with perfect posture and arms anchored to their sides, making no eye contact. It had all the intrigue of a James Bond movie but none of the gadgets and glamour. It was as if we were waiting for 007 to appear. At the time I didn't know it, but the terminal was reserved mostly for government officials. Bob had arranged a private escort through the terminal and onto the plane through top security officials at his job.

I remember being in a state of panic, prior to leaving, asking Bob, "How are we going to get the sample of Taylor's tumor on the plane?" I was thinking of its box marked, "Caution: bio hazardous material." Bob quickly and matter-of-factly responded, "It is taken care of." We were still a synergistic team, and each took on separate responsibilities.

For instance, he knew the tumor was packed in dry ice and couldn't be stored in our luggage. According to the Code of Federal Regulations, "Dry ice (or solid carbon dioxide) is considered a dangerous hazardous material for air transport, and requires special handling." It must never be placed in an airtight container. I had no idea about the catastrophic conditions we could have caused by trying to pass the tumor through our stored luggage. Even if I had known it, I would have never remembered it, given the state I was in. Bob remained strong, stable, and equipped to handle everything or anything.

In a blur, we were quickly escorted onto the plane without passing through security, tumor in hand. We were all set to go, had all our bases covered—or so we thought. We settled comfortably on the plane, and Taylor was calm. As long as she had her oxygen, she felt safe. Jordan was bouncing off the seats, excited about his first trip to Europe. I think half the reason Tales was willing to go was to give Jordan his trip to Germany. How he got to come along is a story unto itself.

Three hours into a nine-hour flight, I checked Taylor's oxygen levels. In complete and utter shock, I realized Taylor had already used up more than half of her oxygen. She was not going to have enough for the entire flight. The fear that overtook my body was the same as one might imagine upon finding out a terrorist was on the plane. In this case, the terrorist was inside Taylor's body, and the mistake was the hospital's miscalculation of the amount of oxygen required.

Earlier that week, I had called the hospital and faxed the required forms that Delta Airlines needed to place oxygen tanks on the plane. Taylor couldn't use the "in case of emergency" drop-down yellow oxygen masks, because they require being able to draw breath from the mask before oxygen comes out, which she was not able to do. Our nurse Jane, one of the most intelligent, hardworking people I have ever met, was not working that day, so I had to work with a different nurse practitioner. I repeated, "Are you sure you checked with the pulmonary department to calculate the liters of oxygen required? Are you sure?" She assured me that she had. I will never know whose mistake it was, hers or the pulmonary department's, but I could never have imagined an error of this magnitude would result.

This mistake caused Taylor the most emotional and physical damage she had ever endured to that point. Umpteen surgeries and dozens of rounds of chemo were no competition. She later told me, "It was the worst day of my life." There is little scarier than feeling like you're suffocating, especially when you're on a plane in the middle of the Atlantic and there's nothing you can do about it.

I slowed down her oxygen. Turning the steel knobs on the tank felt like I was shutting down a faucet to which Taylor's life was tethered. Pure terror emanated from Taylor's face, imploring me to find a solution. With bulging eyes, her skin became as white as paper. She went from shaking, as she gasped for air, to calming down, trying to remain still and reserve her air.

As every mother knows, we can almost literally feel our children's pain. I felt like we were both suffocating. An anesthesiologist was sitting in the row in front of Taylor. I asked him, "Is there anything I can do? Will changing her position to sitting up or lying down help?" He so kindly shook his head no. I can't recall what he looked like, but I can remember his eyes. He acknowledged what I already knew: there was no solution. The only relief came from the small emergency tanks the airliner had onboard for ill passengers. But it wasn't enough.

Many times, over the years, I had offered Taylor one of my lungs, but her answer was always the same: "No. If I get a transplant, I will have to be on anti-rejection drugs, and then I may get cancer again." Now, with a strong determination to continue living, she said, "Mommy, I think I want one of your lungs." Without hesitation, I agreed.

As time elapsed, sheer hysteria set in. I could feel her heart racing, her breathing becoming shallower. Gasping, she said in a voice barely audible, "Promise me, Mommy, I will never again not have enough oxygen to breathe." I made that promise, and I kept it. All I could do was hold on to her hand, try to keep her as calm as possible, and wait out the remaining hours. She did finally doze off for a little while. I thanked God for that enormous gift.

Sixteen years earlier to the exact day of this fateful plane ride, February 16, Taylor was baptized. I clearly remember my mom's words: "Susan, if the girls die before they are baptized, they won't go to heaven." I scoffed at her assertion. How could a new mother possibly think her infant would not go to heaven without the ritual of baptism? I am embarrassed to say that I didn't understand the true meaning of baptism, and I only came to realize it later. The Apostle Paul states: "All of us who were baptized into Christ Jesus were baptized into his death"

(Rom. 6:3,4). I am astounded that exactly sixteen years before that horrible plane ride, Taylor had received the right of passage to eternal life.

When we disembarked in Frankfurt, the paramedics were waiting for us. They briskly escorted Taylor to an urgent care facility in the airport, where she lay for six hours receiving high doses of oxygen to revive her. I wonder, but have never asked, who sent the paramedics. I do know Diana, with the help of top security officials at Bob's firm, had arranged in advance for a team of two Germans to help us while we were there. I don't remember their names, but they were a lovely couple, impeccably dressed, attractive, and knowledgeable. They immediately opened their arms to us. I did not know it at the time, but they had connections on many levels in Germany; we think they both had come from intelligence careers. They were, and still are, mysterious to me.

Once Taylor was stabilized, the German couple arranged for Tales and me to take an ambulance to the little town of Duderstadt, where she was to receive treatment. As the ambulance sped through small town after small town, Taylor lay calmly, never showing any discomfort, as the ambulance bounced along the narrow cobblestone roads. I tried to distract myself by admiring the magnificent, green rolling hills set amongst the quaint towns and homes. But the memories of the prior twenty-four hours relentlessly cut into my heart like a razor. "Mommy, can I text my friends to tell them what happened?" With utter disbelief, I gave her the phone. My girl was back.

How Taylor was able to recover so quickly from a near-death experience, I'll never understand. For the remainder of the ambulance ride, I heard Taylor laughing as the text beeps rolled in one after the other. I marveled at her ability to put terrible things behind her. One way or another, Taylor always seemed to rebound.

Hail Mary

When we arrived at the hotel, I wanted Taylor to take a shower. After the flight she could no longer walk, so I got her into the bathroom by wheelchair. She could not lift her legs over the bathtub. Her frail little body had seen its worst. Determined to please me, she somehow got into the shower. I now question my judgment. Why didn't I rub her down like I had for so many years in the hospital? Was I crazy? I still believed Taylor was okay.

While Taylor was resting, I called Andréa, and in a voice that was barely audible, I implored, "I think you should come to Germany. I don't think we can travel to Vienna. The airplane ride was terrorizing, leaving Tales in a very fragile condition." Andrea cried and, with that, booked a flight to Germany for the next morning.

At the clinic, Taylor's immune cells were removed by way of a machine similar to a dialysis machine. The plan was to combine Taylor's cancer cells with her own immune cells to try to awaken her immune system. Now we had to wait for her cells to multiply. We received the news, "The quality of Taylor's cells is poor, but the quantity is great." The doctor saw this as good news.

Today this type of treatment is available in the United States, but at that time, this physician was considered somewhat of a quack. His theories were considered unfounded and unproven because he was unwilling to submit his theories to controlled trials, which might involve placebos. He merely used the approach, and because it often worked, he attracted more patients. He didn't care about notoriety, just patients. Ironically, the technique and treatment had been pioneered and proven by scientists at Rockefeller University in New York City!

Andrea arrived the next morning in Frankfurt and went outside to the taxi stand, hoping to get someone to drive her to Duderstadt, a few hours away. This was no small task, considering she knew all of two words in German. Several taxis turned her down, but eventually she found some poor soul who agreed.

When she finally arrived, Taylor's eyes lit up. Half laughing, half crying, Andrea told us what happened: "After about an hour and a half riding in the hilly, winding German countryside, I wondered where I was going. I'm pretty sure the driver was thinking the same. Next thing I knew, my cabbie pulled over to talk to some people in a passing car. It felt like a scene out of *The Sound of Music*. The driver began babbling furiously to the passersby in German, and they responded in a very animated way, exclaiming with waving hands, "Duderstadt? *Duderstadt??* Ohhhh! DUDERSTADT!" Then they motioned furiously, indicating it was in a far-off direction."

Taylor was lying in bed listening to Andrea's story, smiling brightly. She seemed to be doing really well that day, having another turnaround. We engaged in conversation about where we'd go on vacation when she was better and we didn't have to pack any medications. Tales interrupted, "You see, Aunt Annie! I told you; I always get better when you come."

That evening we grabbed a bite to eat and prayed the cutting-edge German treatment would work. Before dinner, Corey and Jordan were having difficulty logging on to his computer. The hotel Wi-Fi password contained a German character they couldn't access on his American keyboard. Of course, none of us could figure it out, even with explicit instructions from the front desk—that is, except for Taylor. When she heard about the issue, she grabbed his computer, sighed impatiently, rolled her eyes as if to say, "You're all a bunch of idiots," and effortlessly figured out how to access the German key.

Late that night, Taylor could no longer breathe with the oxygen we had in the hotel. When we called the ambulance, they insisted on taking Taylor to a different hospital about a half hour away, in a town that used to be in East Germany, where most of the people had never learned English. This only added to the surreal nature of the experience. Turns out, though, it also was a godsend. Because none of the healthcare workers spoke English, Taylor remained oblivious to what they were saying about her, especially the conversations about her most recent lung scan.

The next morning Diana went to Andrea's room to wake her up. At the same time, the phone rang, and it was me, dry heaving into the phone. When I finally caught my breath, I said, "It was a really bad night. We were up all night doing chest PT, and she can't breathe. We're in the hospital. Don't tell Diana, but after looking at the most recent scan, the doctors said they expect she has only two days to two weeks." Andrea looked over at Diana, knowing she could hear my voice through the phone. Diana lowered her eyes to the ground, visibly shaken. "I'll meet you at the hospital."

We all prayed for a miracle. We still had that shred of hope that the treatment we had come to Germany for might somehow produce a dramatic reversal of the cancer that was now consuming Taylor's lungs. After all, the oddball German doctor had living patients who had once been in comas when he began treatment and were now many years into remission.

We insisted upon transferring Taylor to a hospital where she could receive the treatment for which we came. In the ambulance I told Taylor, "We are crossing from East Germany to West Germany." She was thrilled that she was personally experiencing a huge part of history by traveling through the place where East and West Germany were reunited.

We finally arrived at the new hospital in Gottingen, where they spoke quite a bit of English. I met Andrea in the waiting room, shaking furiously, whisper screaming, "I'm going to lose my little girl! I'm going to lose my little girl!" I darted into the powder room and violently vomited.

When we went inside to Taylor's room, although her face was half covered by a CPAP breathing apparatus, she was smiling with her eyes and seemed very calm, comfortable, and peaceful. To most people, this would be a life-altering, frightening experience, but to Taylor it was nothing too unusual. She was "breathing" easily, and the sun was shining in through the windows, illuminating the stark-white walls.

She had a notebook on her lap with a pen that allowed her to communicate with us. I rubbed Taylor's arm, lovingly and slowly, and said, "Hi, sweetie. Aunt Annie is here now," in a soothing tone you might use when speaking to a toddler. Taylor impatiently grabbed her pen, frowned, and scribbled, "Why are you speaking to me like I'm an idiot?" Taylor was still Taylor.

Just then Jordan and Corey walked in, and Taylor started an animated conversation via the notebook. Tales was still fully invested in her life and was worried that she had failed Jordan. On her notepad, Taylor wrote to Jordan, "I am sorry." We were all confused until she scribbled, "Remember the paper? That was my fault."

A week before our departure for Germany, Jordan's mother Robbin, Tales, and I were sitting in my room by our glowing fireplace, feeling relaxed. Robbin received a call, clearly became very upset, and left immediately. Taylor could tell from the one-sided exchange of the call that Jordan was in trouble for plagiarizing a paper. She started to cry. I rolled my eyes and said, "His mom will deal with it." Tales blurted out, "You don't understand, Mommy. I wrote that paper, and the teacher is threatening to fail him, which will mean his college acceptance will be revoked! Mommy, I did the research, and I guess while cutting and pasting data I accidentally copied three words, just three words, and his teacher is calling this plagiarizing. I know they are suspicious as to why his grades are all going up, but how could she do this?" Eventually, after much negotiation with the school, his parents got his grade increased to a D on an A-quality paper.

Throughout the afternoon, Taylor was animated, asking Bob, "When will my next scans be?" She then asked if she would be home for Janet's daughter Joanna's sweet sixteen party the following week. Jordan spoke up, boasting, "I was invited, too." Taylor's reaction was so typical. Not only did her facial expressions reveal that she thought his comment was idiotic, but she wrote on the paper, "Duh! That is because Joanna is my friend." Taylor may've been in dire straits, but she never lost her sass, much like my mother had been before we lost her.

While Taylor was with Bob, Andrea and I went to get a cup of coffee in the hospital cafeteria. As we walked, we came across a chapel. I was crying and shaking as we stopped in to pray, telling Andrea, "I want God to take her if she isn't going to last. I don't want my baby to suffer any longer like this." I had never said anything like this before. As she held me in her arms, Andrea remembers thinking, *That's a mother's love. Only a mother would want the best for her child, no matter the cost to herself.*

Later that afternoon, I mumbled, through the severe strain of holding back tears, "You are so special in so many ways, sweetheart." She wanted to know why, raising her hands in the same way she did as a little tot. When Taylor was a baby, when she understood words but before she could speak, I taught her the trick of holding her hands open wide, which meant, "I don't understand." I hadn't seen that gesture in many years, and it nearly tore my heart apart. How could I have ever imagined when I taught her "hands open wide" that she would use that identical symbol years later because her lungs were filled with cancer and she could not speak?

One of Bob's most poignant and most painful moments of the whole odyssey came the night before Taylor died. Taylor took a pen and a piece of paper and asked Bob the same question she had asked over and over again as we moved from doctor to doctor and hospital to hospital over the years: "Daddy, when I go home, what are my next steps? What treatment?" Bob didn't want Tales to see his fear or his eyes well up. With great courage, he looked at her with as much enthusiasm as he could and described two drugs awaiting pediatric trials and an application for a compassionate-use exception to use the drug on a child before trials. She smiled and asked him to write them down. And then she held on to the paper.

Bob sobs, remembering, "It never dawned on Taylor that there would be no next steps or that I wouldn't find them. There were always next steps, and I always had a plan. And right then, I felt a hole in my soul I have never been able to fill. Right then, I knew that I had failed her. I had let her down. I had failed in the most basic responsibility a father has, to keep his kids safe and protect them. It haunts me every day of my life. The hole won't be filled."

The minutes turned into hours, and next thing I knew, it was late at night. The ICU was dark and eerie. Bob and I settled into our "chair-beds," upright, covered in blankets. We hadn't bothered to change our clothes or wash up— nothing new for us.

Tales hugged both Bob and I, one in each arm, and wrote the words, "I'm sorry," on a sheet of paper. I asked Taylor, "Why are you sorry for us?" She simply shrugged her shoulders, indicating we should know how difficult she had made it for us over the last five years. It broke our hearts. Bob and I were *honored* and *privileged* to do anything and everything we could for our precious daughter, at any cost.

When Andrea got back to the new hotel into which they had moved to be closer to the Gottingen hospital, it was almost midnight, very quiet and eerie. The front desk suggested an escort to her room because it was located in a very obscure part of the hotel. Apparently, it was a suite for VIPs who stay at the hotel and want privacy and could house us all. It must've been the work of the German couple again.

Andrea told me, "It seemed like we walked in circles, but when we eventually got to our floor, we walked down a long hallway. I remember looking at the small, thin grey metal numbers on the doors as we approached our room. Room number 600, 602, 604, and so on. Next thing you know, we were at the end of the hallway, the room just before ours being number 634. Upon reaching our room, I thanked my escort and looked up. I was standing before a massive brown wooden door, fitting of a VIP suite, and on it were huge numbers: 666."

Losing Taylor

Taylor woke Bob up, telling him, "I have to go to the bathroom." He got the bedpan and looked at her numbers on the hospital monitors. Taylor went right back to sleep, but Bob woke me, speaking in between sobs, "Taylor's numbers are plummeting. It's only a matter of minutes or seconds before the ICU nurses will come in." In some sort of out-of-body experience, I quickly asked for Taylor to be put on heavy medications so she would not awaken and know she was dying.

They complied, but in typical Taylor fashion, she broke through the medications. "Taylor's awake!" I screamed, racing out into the hallway. "That's impossible," responded one of the ICU nurses. "Come and see, then!" The nurses entered the room as perplexed as we were. With composure I never knew I had, I asked, "Taylor, my sweetheart, do you want more meds? Are you in pain?" She shook her hand in an all-too-familiar fashion, indicating she was feeling "so-so."

That was the last time either Bob or I spoke to a responsive Taylor. Just recently I was telling this to a friend who never knew Taylor's story, and she said to me, "Of course Taylor broke through the pain meds. She had to see her mommy and daddy one more time."

With each hour, her breathing got shallower, and even in her sleep, with morphine easing her way to the light, her little body struggled to breathe. At some point, the German doctors convinced me that I needed to be talking to Taylor, forcefully insisting that she could hear me. "Hold her hand; sit next to her; talk to her," asserted the heavily accented German doctor. I looked at the clock. It was half past three in the morning. I slumped in my chair.

The doctor peered in through the faded and cracked glass that separated us from him. He caught my eye and frowned. I looked at the clock. Time was passing so slowly and yet too quickly. Later, in an even sterner voice, he said again, "You must talk to her, or at least hold her hand." I looked at the clock ticking away, another minute, another hour, but I could hardly move.

A change in shift brought in new doctors. "Keep on talking to her; climb into bed with her; she can hear you." Again, they insisted Taylor could hear me and listening to my voice would be very comforting to her. Again, I looked at the clock and wondered why I was keeping track of the time.

By about five, I called Andrea. She immediately arrived with some food she had pilfered from the hotel buffet wrapped in napkins and tried to get us to eat something. She asked Bob if it was okay to stay. He assured her it was, giving Andrea a huge, loving hug. I was completely listless, unable to really converse with Tales. We all sat there, just staring at Taylor, waiting.

Finally, I put on Taylor's favorite red hat, a wool knit hat with a pom-pom on the top and bottom of each tassel that, by any rational measure, was just plain goofy looking. The hat looked so ridiculous that whenever Taylor wore it, most people burst into uproarious laughter. Bill called it an "automatic insanity defense" hat. Taylor, more so than the others, found it particularly hilarious whenever I put it on and used to say I looked like Waldo, a character from one of her favorite childhood books. For some unknown reason, donning this silly hat helped me snap out of my emotionally induced coma and in a perverse way gave me the strength I so desperately needed to become both emotionally and physically ambulatory again.

Like a shadow in the night, I stood up and purposefully walked across the dimly lit, unforgiving hospital room toward my beautiful baby girl lying motionless in her bed, very close to death. With bulging eyes, tangled hair, tattered clothes, and that red hat, I got into bed with Taylor. I pulled my baby's warm body close to me, and with tears drenching both of us, I stroked Taylor's hair, took in her scent, and studied her beautiful hands and toes for the last time.

I desperately tried to commit to memory, for all eternity, every unique and exquisite facet of Taylor's face and body. I tried to summon the strength to speak to her one last time as the cacophony of the various machines and monitors clanged and clattered, taunting me with every startling beep. My lips and body quivered uncontrollably as I finally spoke: "I love you; I love you—don't leave me here alone. You are all things great in this world. I need you. Please, please don't leave me, my perfect angel. How will I ever live without you? Why can't you live the life you love so much? Why? I am so sorry, my baby."

As the time passed, my head was spinning, while I lost any sense of the conscious world. Taylor and I were in our world. The day before I had asked her, "Do you want a towel wrapped around your head? The CPAP is blowing very cold air." Taylor responded in writing, "No, the cold air makes me breathe easier." A year or so after Taylor passed away, I was speaking to a psychic who told me Taylor was telling her, "Mommy, you were right, I was cold. I needed my red hat."

By mid-morning, the German doctor from Duderstadt arrived at the hospital with a shot containing the experimental treatment that we had come for in the first place. "Should I give it to her?" inquired the doctor to Bob. Bob's eyes welled with tears. "Yes," he said, tentatively and softly, as his voice was cracking. As he slowly lifted his eyes, he became surer of his answer. A little louder, he said, "I promised her the other day that she would get it, no matter what, so yes." The doctor nodded and injected Taylor's motionless arm.

Beata saved us again by arranging for us to meet, through her mother's long-time connection in Poland, a loving and adoring priest. He had visited Taylor days earlier while she still could converse with him. Taylor was so touched that Beata had made this possible. She had always been unstoppable, but how she located a priest in the tiny town of Duderstadt, corresponded with him, and arranged for us to meet him seemed beyond any mortal's capability. She is the definition of pure love. Out of nowhere on this last day, he arrived to give Taylor her last rites.

I always worried about how Taylor would receive her last rites, because we never wanted to tell her she might be dying. Thankfully, not only was she in a medically induced state of sleep but also her last rites were given to her in German. Even if she could hear, she would have never understood. Beata gave me the greatest gift a mother could receive while her daughter was dying. I am forever grateful to her, not only for this but also for all the love she gave my family and all the sacrifices she made over five long years. I couldn't have done it without her.

I'm not sure how the ensuing hours passed as I continued to speak with Taylor. I saw on the monitor that Taylor's heart was beating furiously, almost as if she was running a race. Was she trying to tell us she was sprinting, just as she had done her whole life?

The doctors insisted we bring Corey to the hospital, but we were very hesitant. We finally agreed, and both Corey and Jordan came. Within minutes of their arrival, Taylor's pulse began racing, and her oxygen climbed for the last time. We all huddled together, holding each other tightly, encircling Taylor, and bellowed our favorite chorus from the song written for her so long ago: "Everything's okay if I'm with Tay!" Those may've been the last words she ever heard. She took that moment, surrounded by her loved ones, to move on to everlasting life, leaving us alone without her shining spirit. I believe Tales waited for Corey because she wanted to see her one last time and needed her help to go to heaven.

The doctor came in and shut off the machines. All was quiet for a moment. Everything was still. She slipped away with Bob's hand on hers. Bob felt that she was gone, but she was still there. He cried. It just came, and it wouldn't stop. No wailing or screaming. It was just an immense and profound sadness.

Our love story continued almost immediately after Taylor's passing. Sobbing, I held my beautiful angel for that last time and stroked her hair. As I glided my hand over her soft cotton pillowcase, a little heart soldered to the charm bracelet I was wearing broke off. I stared at the shiny, silver heart against the backdrop of the white pillowcase in utter disbelief. At the time, I thought of it as a symbol of my forever broken heart, but now I believe that she was telling me that although we were physically separated on this earth, we would never be separated spiritually. She was taking my heart with her.

In silence, we all said goodbye to Tales. When it was Bob's time, he kissed her cheek and embraced her. He said, "I could feel sweat at her temple. And it dawned on me that she fought to the very end. She never quit. Taylor didn't lose her battle; she just ran out of time." Bob also told Taylor how sorry he was. Digging deep, he told her, "I'm sorry I let you down. Sorry I made so many mistakes along the way of your treatment. I hope you can forgive me." I will never understand or comprehend why Bob thinks he let her down. The thought of it breaks my heart.

We were escorted to a waiting room; I guess it was so we wouldn't disturb other patients. Abruptly, Bob stood up and went back into her room by himself. "I needed to say one more thing to her and feel her one more time. I walked back as quickly as I could so that I wouldn't be too late before they took her away. She was still there, lying peacefully. I leaned over to kiss her and to whisper in her ear. For all the time I had spent apologizing that I had let her down, I had forgotten to say, 'I love you.'"

We lost Taylor on February 22, 2008. It was a day filled with a heartbreak I cannot put into words. My body went limp, the tears would not stop, and all I could do was stare at the sky, looking for my baby, but really thinking that when I returned to her hospital room, there would be my bright and cheerful Taylor. Reality would not set in for many years. In many ways, it still has not.

We had to tell Ryan, who was a continent away. She was in her nine o'clock Italian class when we first tried to call. After class, when she saw the missed call, she had a horrible sense of foreboding and called us back immediately. With heart-wrenching sobs, Corey told her—she had insisted that she be the one to tell Ryan. "My immediate reaction was that she was joking," Ryan told us later. "Not in a funny way but in that it couldn't be true, and in the span of what was probably only a few seconds, I went through tons of scenarios that could explain why Corey would say Taylor died, but none of them made sense."

Ryan was only eighteen. How could we give her this news without being there? I took the phone from Corey and asked Ryan to walk to her friend Hannah's room and stay there until Janet arrived. I had already called Janet in the middle of the night, barely able to speak, and told her, "I'm losing my baby!" Screaming and sobbing, she said, "I will get on the earliest flight I can to be with Ryan."

When Ryan heard the same news from me she had heard from her sister, that was the moment she understood and lost control. All I heard were Ryan's shrieking screams and wailing, the most horrifying screams I have ever heard and which I will never forget. At some point, I do remember Hannah saying to me, "Don't worry, Mrs. Matthews. I will take care of Ryan."

We found out later that day that the German couple had arranged to file papers with the German Consulate that morning, stating Taylor had already passed away. It was a Friday, and if the papers were not filed that morning, the Consulate wouldn't have been able to sign them until Monday, which would've prohibited Taylor from leaving the country until then. At the same time, Diana was arranging for a private plane to take everyone back home. Apparently, it could take up to two weeks to bring Taylor home on a commercial flight. All we knew was that we desperately needed to get back to Ryan in the United States.

Andrea called Bill to tell him we lost Taylor. Samantha was crushed. Even though Sammie was so young, the depth of their relationship was somehow enormous. It's as if they understood each other on a level that the rest of us couldn't comprehend. They were as close as two cousins could be, despite a ten-year age gap. Actually, it was the same age gap as between Andrea and myself, two souls similarly intertwined for all of eternity.

Moments after Uncle Bill told Samantha that Taylor had died, a plate that was hanging on their kitchen wall came crashing down onto the counter. Oddly, this is not uncommon in our family. Many times, when a family member dies, something falls off a wall, telling us sometimes before we even get the call. Samantha, together with Bill, cried until there were no more tears left. Then Samantha furrowed her brow and said she would always remember Taylor as her "Sleeping Beauty," a tribute to Samantha's then-favorite fairy tale depicting a sixteen-year-old princess who falls into a deep slumber.

The next morning, Samantha told Bill she saw Taylor in what she called a "daydream" just before she woke up. She blurted out, "Taylor looked like she was in a bubble. Her hair was still short, but she was not sick anymore."

"What did Taylor say?"

"Nothing."

"Then how did you know she wasn't sick anymore?"

"I don't know; I just do," was all she could muster. If a six-year-old were going to make up a story, it would be fraught with hyperbole and tied with a bow. Its simplicity spoke volumes.

In a trance, we somehow made it to the hotel VIP suite together. We felt like Taylor was still with us, but the reality was, she was not. Numb, I called Taylor's name several times, not fully understanding why she didn't respond. Corey was trying to be so brave, but she looked at me with tear-filled eyes and said, "Mommy, are you going to be okay?"

"Yes, I am, Corey," I said, holding her in my arms, surprising even myself that I could answer coherently. "Because I have you." I don't recall much more except that the comfort and warmth of Corey's embrace literally saved me in that moment, and together with Ryan and Bob, they continue to save me today. I have no idea what happened for the remainder of the night or if I even slept.

I am immensely grateful that Andrea was with us. Taylor was extremely close to my sister and her family, and the love Andrea's family shared with us has kept us standing. People often ask me why I am not upset that I don't have a relationship with Lynn. My answer is and will always be, "I'm so lucky to have the love of my life in Andrea. We are soul mates, and I don't need anyone else."

The next day, before we returned to the States, I prayed, asking Tales to send me a second sign. In Frankfurt, while waiting for our flight, we walked aimlessly across the icy, bone-chilling streets in a state of complete confusion. We entered a quaint outdoor square where a small band was playing German folk tunes, and suddenly, they began singing, in English, the Beatles' song "Let it Be." And in that moment, Mother Mary spoke words of wisdom to me, too. Although no song or words or poetry, no matter how beautiful, will ever make life without her okay, it felt enormously comforting to get a sign from Taylor right away. Some may call it a coincidence, but I call it a wink.

What Do I Have to Be Angry About?

Father Tony, Bill's dearest friend who is a Catholic priest, presided over Taylor's funeral mass. He profoundly told us, "Taylor's life, however short, had a beginning, a middle, and an end. Although her life was a novelette rather than a novel, it was complete." I found his words comforting, but at the same time, to my mortal ears, her life seems to have been abruptly cut short.

Now, after years of soul searching for answers via therapists, ministers, priests, rabbis, mediums, books, and research, I have come to realize that Taylor was here for only a short time to teach us the lesson that love is the most powerful force and that it is all we need to live. She wanted nothing more than to give and receive love. Three weeks prior to her passing, I asked, Taylor, again. "Why are you not angry that you are tied to an oxygen tank, missing school and your friends?" She replied, "Mommy, what do I have to be angry about? Everyone loves me."

At Taylor's funeral, I wanted the Beatles' song "All You Need is Love" to be played in church. It embodied everything that Taylor's life had been about. What was I thinking? This was the Catholic Church. They forbade it, but in true Taylor spirit, our plans would not be thwarted. After the mass, as we proceeded out of the church, despite their rules, we, along with hundreds of others, bellowed the lyrics to "All You Need Is Love." I know Taylor was watching and laughing, as it was a prank she would have planned herself and a song she adored.

Corey's confirmation was less than four weeks after we lost Taylor. As we talked about her upcoming day, she screamed, "Taylor promised me she would be here!" I dug deep in my soul, my eyes burning but refusing to well up, and answered, "Taylor wanted to be here, sweetheart." That seemed to make it worse. There was no way to console Corey.

On a bitterly cold day, in late afternoon, Ryan, Corey, and I headed out to have an invitation printed for the confirmation. "Evites" did not yet exist. I had always had beautiful printed invitations for all my girls' special days, and this would be no exception.

We decided to go to a different stationery store than normal to avoid bumping into anyone we knew. We walked into the store and began perusing samples of invitations. Suddenly Ryan gasped, "Mommy! Corey! Look at this one!" Her voice was piercing, and we ran over to see what was up.

Ryan had found a sample invitation that read as follows:

We proudly & lovingly announce the birth of
Our little angel ("little angel" rather than "daughter")
Taylor Anne (spelled exactly the same way)
February 22 (the date of her passing)
9 lbs. 11 ounces (symbolizing her premonition of 9/11)
22 inches

I believe Taylor was telling me she had been reborn an angel. Samantha would say it was God sending the sign, but either way, it gives me great comfort. Sometimes my sanity is maintained believing that Taylor is now an angel and that someday, over the rainbow, I will see her again.

I quickly asked the cashier, with tears streaming, "Can we have this invitation?" Clearly, she had no clue as to why I was crying, nor did she understand the importance of it. She answered, "I can make a copy," to which I responded sadly, "That would be fine." I had the copy laminated and, together with very special photographs of all three of my girls, have placed it in a "Taylor blue" leather envelope. There is no bag too small for this envelope. I carry it everywhere. I don't believe it was a coincidence that Taylor left us on February 22 (2/22) as she was born on November 1 (11/1). She loved numbers and will always be my little mathematician!

On the day of Corey's confirmation, I have no idea how I found the strength to enter the church where Taylor's funeral had been just a few short weeks prior. It was our church: Bob and I were married there, Corey's baptism was there, and, as of that day, all three of my girls would be confirmed there. I was determined to be present for Corey, but I knew I would never enter those doors again after her confirmation. In the end, my love for Corey transcended my pain, and I was able to be there for her. She certainly deserved it.

The reality is that I was not physically or emotionally present for Ryan and Corey for five long years, during very fragile and formative years of their lives. I couldn't address their adolescent issues, their homework, their hopes, their dreams, or their fears. In the ways that count most, they were all alone, treading icy waters after falling off the Titanic, and their only life rafts were Andrea and Bill, Beata, my parents, and my dearest friends. As wonderful as they all were, no one can take the place of a parent. When a child is diagnosed with cancer, its poisonous lesions engulf and scar the entire family.

The truth is, if Taylor hadn't been the sick child, I'm not sure she would've taken it as well as her sisters did. From birth she *demanded* my attention, and she certainly had much less patience than Ryan and Corey. Many times, her sisters gave in because they couldn't deal with the drama or aggravation. Had Taylor been left home alone for five years, she would've pitched a fit daily.

Even given their calm temperaments, it truly amazes me that Ryan and Corey were willing and able to sacrifice so much. Their love for Taylor and our whole family was so powerful that, in the face of crisis, they didn't crumble. Each fought to keep everything together. They never "acted out" or told us they were angry, but I imagine they were. It would be only natural when Taylor got 99 percent of my attention. Instead, they desperately tried to make everything ideal, telling us, "We didn't want you to have more problems."

To a fault, they still strive to make things perfect for Bob and me. They are wildly concerned about my well-being, and to this day, they become distraught if they think I am angry with them or that they didn't do the right thing. Their impulse to be "the best" still remains with them today. I wish I could change their feelings, but instead I can only validate them. They come from a place of love. Even though I tell them how grateful I am for them, a trillion times wouldn't be enough.

I wish I could fill in all the blanks during the years after we lost Taylor and remember how we found each other again, but I recall very little. Bob quit his job to stay home with us. He held us up, literally and figuratively, sacrificing himself while grieving tremendously, to help us. I know I would not be the person I am without him. I remember moments from that time period, like when Ryan sprained her ankle, when we traveled to Turkey, and definitely when I lost friends on purpose, but I cannot recall details about each of our emotional well-being. I do know we surrounded each other with everlasting and unconditional love, the most powerful force, which kept us together as a family. Somehow, we survived. Today Bob and I are so proud of what Ryan and Corey have been able to achieve. Ryan graduated from Wake Forest University and Corey from Cornell University, and both are now working in New York City. Each of them are very different, yet much the same as well.

If anyone is an old soul, it's Ryan. Looking back, she was born with the kind of patience and understanding one usually only achieves after gaining life experience. Simultaneously, she has always been extremely young at heart and playful. Andrea says Ryan is "true north." True north is the direction that goes straight to the North Pole, and it's different from "magnetic north," which can change according to circumstances. Ryan is "true north" because her internal moral compass doesn't change direction based on society's or anyone else's standards. She's solid and steady, like a rock, and you can count on her to do the right thing. She cares for others with great compassion and is as beautiful on the inside as she is on the out. She is also extremely proud and resourceful, a trait perhaps she didn't always have but had to adopt quickly when she overnight became the head of the household and Corey's caregiver.

Today, Corey is tall, beautiful, and elegant, with long, thick brown hair and eyelashes to match. She is very independent, outgoing, fun loving, and has always taken great pride in her academics. She cares deeply for her friends and family, going out of her way to help others, particularly when they are in trouble, with great empathy and concern. She will gladly stay behind from any social gathering to help a friend in need. Corey has a heart of gold and grit to match. She takes on seemingly impossible tasks with ease and dedication. If she loves you, you will know it. Taylor certainly did. The shine in her eyes will always consist, partially, of a reflection of both of her older sisters.

We strive every day to help Ryan and Corey live life as normally as possible, and they have succeeded. Bob and I will never fully recover, but Taylor's sisters have to, and it is what Taylor would want and expect from them. If she could voice her opinion, I'm sure it would be, "Go on living, loving, learning, and experiencing everything you can from life. And most of all, have fun!" Doing so doesn't mean that her memory is forgotten. If anything, doing what Taylor would want is a nod to her memory more than any other gesture would or could be.

Today, I cry every time I hear Ryan tell me, "You are an amazing mother, and I am fine—actually I am good—and that is in large part because of how you took care of me as best you could." Corey says with amazement, "I am astounded that you and Daddy were able to step up and find ways to be there for us emotionally and physically after all you've been through."

But, it is I who is the most astounded. In the face of horrific tragedy, we remain a family.

I Hope You're Dancing in the Sky

Every day, Taylor's absence is evident, but her presence is felt. In her memory, on the one-year anniversary of her passing, we decided to gather up her family and friends for a celebration of her life. It was excruciating, but it was something we had to do to honor her strength, courage, and spirit. My memory of that evening fades in and out like the tide, rolling in with a vengeance and then, with equal intensity, rushing out with the undertow.

The event took place on a biting, windy February night, when icy temperatures froze the streets. The weather perfectly reflected our states of mind: turbulent, gloomy, and bitterly cold. Piles of snow and ice mocked us everywhere, promising to remain for at least another month. I still wasn't sure if this was a nightmare from which I would soon awaken, and I often still feel that way; I probably always will.

As we walked inside the Scarsdale Woman's Club, where Taylor's memorial was being held, we were immediately soothed by the sharp contrast of its warm ambiance. The room was aglow with soft, golden light from flickering candles atop golden silk sheers and burgundy tablecloths, enveloping us like a comfy blanket. The aroma of coffee and an assortment of sweet and tangy desserts, the kind that melt in your mouth, was a sensory celebration.

I remember wearing a pretty white dress covered with red roses. I had to go shopping, one of my least favorite activities, as a year later I was still a good forty pounds above my normal weight. During the last few years of Taylor's illness, the pounds had piled on, due to the elevated stress hormones that had infiltrated my bloodstream.

As I stood up to speak, Bob sat right next to me, holding me up. He winked, assuring me all would be okay. I nervously scanned the room, looking from face to face, hoping that my words might give Taylor's friends closure. My body began to shake, and my nervous habit of playing with my hair caused me to realize that my palms were sweating. I fought against my own body, willing myself to not give in to my nerves. I had to be brave like Taylor and for Taylor.

I caught the eye of one of Taylor's dearest friends, Becca. They were always there for each other and would defend the other, no matter the issue. I smiled to myself, remembering the night Becca came over pissed about someone and plopped herself down in the middle of the bed between Tales and Jordan, for friendly advice from both the female and male perspective. I'm not sure how Jordan reacted, but Taylor was furious. Half naked, in just a long T-shirt and flip flops, Tales stormed out of the house to a party conveniently located right across the street and had it out with the person with whom Becca was upset. Both the outfit and the conversation were one for the record books. This vibrant memory held me up.

I began,

I want to thank all of you for gathering tonight to celebrate both Taylor's life and all of your lives. Thank you for sharing your life with Taylor and for showering her with gifts of love, laughter, friendship, and support, and for being Taylor's buddies in her never-ending adventures. We also want to thank Taylor's teachers and Nancy, for your never-ending support, compassion, and empathy for Taylor's situation and for creating an environment where she could fulfill her passion for learning while dealing with a serious illness.

So where do I begin? Taylor came into our lives and left way too quickly. If she could, she would turn over heaven and earth to be here tonight. I hope you can all feel her presence in your hearts, tonight and always. You left footprints in her heart and nothing can ever change that. As her parents, the words 'thank you' could never begin to express how Bob and I feel. We are so blessed to have watched Taylor live a happy, fun, and fulfilled life with the people who meant the most to her: her sisters, her family, her friends, and her teachers. All of you gave Taylor the gift of love. You see, for Taylor, she could deal with her diagnosis and all the treatments. What she wanted was to live. As you all know, boisterous times at our house were countless and precious.

As Tales got older, many times, our home hosted crazy pool nights where, no matter what, the boys threw the girls into the pool with their cell phones in hand. The pool was usually filled with as many as twenty kids, laughing like crazy till all hours of the night, while the hot tub was filled to the brim.

When I reflect back on Taylor's life, I remember how important and cherished her life in school, both elementary and high school, was. My mind often wanders right into the classrooms of Edgemont, and I find myself crying when I think about what the teachers at EHS and Nancy gave of themselves to my angel. All of you imparted important life lessons, not just about academics; you taught Tales much more than a textbook ever could. You recognized her zest and passion for learning, and she knew you were 100 percent behind her. She never took the gift of learning or the gift of her teachers and advisors for granted. She recognized your special calling in life, a calling to work with children. You made school a stress-free and enriching place for Taylor and, very importantly, respected Taylor and let her express herself.

I am struggling for words. I hope you understand that this was written from my heart. I wish I had overhead projectors where I could show you, in bold, what my heart wants you to so badly understand. You not only loved her but you helped her. Many times, Taylor was not willing to accept help, but you managed to give it to her through your acts of pure love. Whenever you face any kind of challenge in your life, remember what she would tell you: LIFE SUCKS; WEAR A HELMET!

We can never prepare ourselves for the loss of a friend and a sister. We all miss her terribly, but I truly believe she would want all of you to hold her in your hearts and, at the same time, to move forward, be happy, go to college, enjoy life to the fullest, do things for her that she never got to do, and live to your heart's passion. Do whatever excites you. Live with purpose and excitement. Believe in yourself; believe you can do anything because, if you try, you can. Shower others with the love you showered Tales with and truly make your daily life an adventure. And lastly, cherish your friends and your family as if your life depended on it. Because always remember in life: if you have love, you have everything.

Goodbyes are not forever. Goodbyes are not the end. They simply mean we will miss you until we meet again. We love you with our entire heart, sweet angel.

Somewhere over the Rainbow

I think about Taylor every day of my life. Sometimes I touch my belly, trying to remember Taylor's little movements when I was pregnant with her—a time when the miracle of Taylor was growing inside me, a time when our emotional bond and unconditional love was seared together forever, a time when I would dream about holding my little one, and a time when God first graced me with the blessing of being her mother.

I gave birth to my angel, and I will always be Taylor's mother. Death cannot rob me of that.

I am and will always be a mother of three girls, and together we will always be a family of five. No person or force of nature can ever take that away.

Taylor left our family with so many lessons. Many times, my thoughts return to a poem she wrote just a few months before her passing, entitled "The World Is Just Not Black and White."

Red, orange, yellow, green, blue, purple, or pink, colors of my life, colors of me
A color to celebrate with, one to cry with and a color for everything in between.
White, white for everything pure and whole.

Black. For when there is no other color to feel
Black. It's called darkness for a reason
Black. The color of the inside of my eyelids as I fall asleep wishing I won't wake up
Black. Covering everything else, one shade one true color
Black. As the paint covers the rainbow of my life, trickling slowly like blood.
Black. Cold metal, cold water, cold hands
Black. As the room blinks in front of my eyes
Black. As voices fade and everything leaves
Black. As I forget, as I take a deep breath
But then it's not so black, because there is always tomorrow

Red, orange, yellow, green, blue, purple, or pink, colors of my life, colors of me
A color to celebrate with, one to cry with and a color for everything in between.
White, white for everything pure and whole.
White. The first thing I see as I wake up.
White. The color of making it through.
White. Remembering, recognizing,
White. Knowing where you've been and where you're going
White. The peace of a blank canvas.
White. Faces, faces and voices coming back to me
White. The last minute for me to grab only me

White. The Last color before the colors of life start to come back

Red, orange, yellow, green, blue, purple, or pink, colors of my life, colors of me
A color to celebrate with, one to cry with and a color for everything in between.

Most of all, Taylor taught us that during every dark moment, there's a brighter day in the future, and for every black day, there's a rainbow. So, in the meantime:

Paint your hair blue.

Go on that midnight ice cream run.

Break the rules.

Dance in the rain.

And never forget to say I love you.

It's only fitting that Taylor be the one to help get us through our grief.

The Gold at the End of the Rainbow:

The Taylor Matthews Foundation

Taylor left me with her legacy, the torch of her mission, tay-bandz, whose name has been changed to the Taylor Matthews Foundation. Her wishes, hopes, and dreams give great meaning and purpose to my life. As I awaken every morning and think about Taylor, I am reminded of why what I do to continue her work is so important. Today we are keeping Taylor's spirit, her thirst to make change, and her dedication to help others alive.

Today, we have raised hundreds of thousands of dollars for pediatric cancer research. We have funded research at Columbia University Medical Center, MD Anderson Cancer Center, the National Institute of Health, and Memorial Sloan Kettering. We are embarking on a new day in pediatric cancer: a day of less toxic and more successful treatments, greater hope for sick children and their families, and easier access to therapies of all kinds. We are a few steps closer to achieving Taylor's mission that all children with cancer will live long, healthy, productive lives. Our research is saving lives today.

Taylor's mission has now made its way to Washington, DC. We actively lobby childhood cancer legislation on behalf of all the voiceless children with cancer. When Corey was with us in DC, she eloquently explained to members of Congress and their aides:

"I was only eight years old when my sister was diagnosed with cancer. At a very young age, I was exposed to tragedy and the terrible illness that took my sister's life. I know it firsthand. I've grown up angry—that I couldn't save my sister, that she was taken from me, and that there are countless other young siblings who will lose their sisters and brothers. I don't want other children to suffer and lose their battle to cancer. I have a responsibility to learn all that I can, influence others, and make this country a better place for those who live here. I was a few months shy of being fourteen when I watched my sister die, and there was nothing my parents or I could do. I want to have an impact. It is unconscionable to think that the government refuses to make childhood cancer a priority."

Corey continued by highlighting the inadequacy and unfairness of the health-care system. Corey's words rang through the hallways of the Senate and House of Representatives. She is making a difference for her sister who cannot.

Taylor didn't live long enough to know that in recognition of tay-bandz's donations to Columbia, a sarcoma lab was dedicated to her, one in which her cousin Samantha recently interned. In a magnificent ceremony, where again I found myself standing in for Taylor, Corey held me up as we cut a huge white ribbon opening the doors to the lab. A silver plaque to the left of the entrance is engraved with the words, "Funding for research made possible by Taylor Matthews and tay-bandz."

Her story continues. There will never be a period at its end

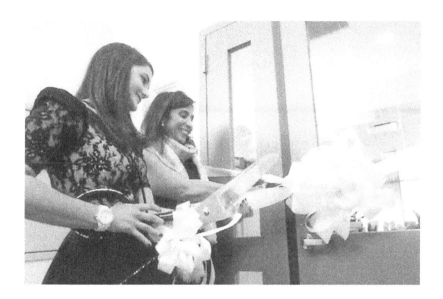

Treatment Tips

In the course of Taylor's cancer journey, we gathered many "nuggets of gold," or anecdotal lessons, through the trial and error of treatment. If you or a loved one is going through a long illness, you may find some of these tips helpful. Naturally, I am writing from the perspective of a parent of a cancer patient; however, many of these tips can be applied to a variety of situations and illnesses.

The information provided is not a substitute for medical or professional care, and you should not use this information in place of a visit, consultation, or the advice of your physician or other healthcare provider. It is based on my experience and should be used for educational purposes only.

Diagnosis

1. Send your pathology to other hospitals to confirm diagnosis and to analyze the tumor. Your hospital will send the slides for you for a nominal fee.

2. Get a second, third, and even fourth opinion! Bring copies of your scans to the doctor providing the second opinion or mail in advance if a second opinion is discussed over the phone. Do not count on your hospital to send it.

3. Research your disease. Many doctors will warn you that much of the information on the web is inaccurate, contradictory, generalized, and overwhelming. If you can put the fear factor aside, the Internet can be very helpful in explaining different treatment options, identifying

215

current research, and citing the names of doctors and institutions where valuable support can be found.

4. Ask your doctors to collaborate with the doctors at other institutions, which will give you the best treatment options available nationally or globally.

5. Many medical terms may be foreign. Continue to ask if you don't understand a term used or understand what the doctors are saying. No question is a bad one!

6. Have your tumor analyzed as soon as possible by Precision Medicine. Precision Medicine uses genomic profiling to make personalized, genetically informed treatment recommendations and assist with clinical decision making, culminating in better outcomes for patients. When the biopsy is performed, a sample can be taken for this purpose.

7. You will receive your protocol (treatment plan) and a timeline. The timeline most likely will change based upon low blood counts. Have a doctor or nurse explain in detail what the numbers mean in a complete blood count (CBC) so you can watch your numbers and spot trends.

8. If you do not understand your protocol, ask if there is a summary of the protocol available for your review.

9. You will most likely need a central line under your skin (a Broviac or a port) because chemotherapy is very difficult to administer through an IV, and over time, your veins will not hold up. Determine with your doctors whether a Broviac or a port is most suitable. If it is for your child, do consider his or her choice.

10. Ask about immunology treatment options.

11. Consider harvesting your stem cells. They can be used later to rescue your immune system. Sometimes your immune system can stay low for an extended period of time, leaving you at high risk for infection. Infusion of your own stem cells will bring back your immune system quickly. When harvesting, make sure your stem cells are frozen in small packages so you can use them several times.

Scans

1. Insist on getting results from scans immediately. Some hospitals will tell you results may take days. Don't accept that answer. Every moment waiting for test results is grueling.

2. When booking scans, do not accept a scan appointment later in the day. You cannot eat before a scan and will be very uncomfortable.

3. Do not take any narcotics before your scans, because narcotics on an empty stomach can cause extreme nausea.

4. Get a copy of every radiology report and read it in depth. Don't let your doctors summarize it. Sometimes they tell you only what they want you to hear.

5. Get a copy of the disc from every scan (MRI, PET, CT, bone scan, X-ray, ECHO, EKG, etc.).

Medications

1. Check all medications and chemotherapy you receive. Anyone can dispense wrong medications by accident. Trust your doctors, but check them every step of the way—it can only help!

2. Both at home and in the hospital, keep a log of your medications and the time they were dispensed. Phone apps can help you with this.

3. Research your chemotherapy and medications. The doctors will require you to sign reams of paper that likely will explain frightening side effects. You will feel more comfortable if you understand beforehand the medication/chemotherapy you are getting.

4. If anything seems wrong, call your nurse and/or your doctor immediately. Trust your gut!

5. Whether in the ICU or inpatient, pain management doctors will decide what pain medications to administer. Do not accept what they say if your pain is not manageable. You will quickly know what works best for you.

6. Check the results of all of your blood counts. Ask for and maintain copies of everything, and if anything seems unusual, bring it to your medical professional's attention.

7. A side effect of chemotherapy and pain medications is constipation. Address the problem before it happens.

8. Get an Insuflon, which is a small access point put into your leg that needs to be changed about once a week. This way, you can give yourself a shot at home, and it won't be painful. When inserting an Insuflon or accessing a port, ask for Emla cream (numbing cream).

9. Seek alternative treatments, such as acupuncture and massage, to alleviate nausea and pain.

10. If you overdose on any of your medications, even if you seem to be fine, do contact your physician immediately.

Urgent Situations

Call your doctor immediately if you are experiencing anything unusual. No question is a bad one.

Emergency Room Visits

1. Before leaving for the ER, call your on-call doctor and advise them of the problem. Make sure that your doctor calls the ER to tell them you are en route and that because you have cancer you cannot be subjected to other sick people in the waiting room.

2. Upon arrival, insist upon immediate attention.

Surgery

1. Seek second opinions and different surgical options.

2. Speak to your personal anesthesiologist on the day of your surgery. Don't count on your pre-op anesthesiologist to pass along information.

3. If you have an allergy, make sure you are wearing a red wristband and discuss the allergy with the anesthesiologist.

4. Many people become nauseated after general anesthesia. Ask for an intravenous infusion of anti-nausea drugs before you wake up.

5. If your child is the one receiving surgery, insist on going into the operating room until he or she receives anesthesia.

6. Ask for updates during surgery to alleviate stress, especially if surgery exceeds the amount of time you expected (which often happens).

7. Insist on being in the recovery room when your child or loved one wakes up. It is very frightening for your child to wake up without a loved one nearby.

Family and Friends

1. Family and friends want to help, but often do not know what to do except send gifts and meals. Let them know these are helpful! A great gift you can ask for is for them to give blood and platelets and reserve them for your child. Never accept "pooled platelets" (platelets from several donors), which can cause an allergic reaction. You want platelets from a single donor.

2. Family and friends can be apprehensive to pry but often want an update. A popular and unobtrusive way to provide this is for you to write a blog. Not only is it cathartic to do so, it is also a relatively easy way for you to control the information available about your situation. It also removes the pressure of having to return calls and emails. You can easily create a blog through the website caringbridge.org.

3. Ask your family and friends to visit as often as feasible.

The most important thing you can do in this journey is to trust your gut instincts. Doctors can sometimes make you feel like your questions are insignificant, stupid, or a waste of time. Do not blindly trust anyone. That is not to say you should distrust your physicians; on the contrary, in many ways, they are your lifelines. However, they are just as human as anyone else, and you have a right to advocate for yourself or your loved one at all costs. Do what is right for your family and remember every day is a gift. Enjoy it! Cancer is not a death sentence. In many ways, it provides an eye-opening opportunity to live your life to the fullest. That's what Taylor did. That's what she taught me, and that is what she would want you to know.

Acknowledgments

To the many heroes in Taylor's life, I will forever be grateful. She felt secure, safe, and supported by all your love, compassion, and the limitless hours you spent helping her.

To all those who never knew Taylor, you have continued to keep her alive by reading her story. Thank you!

I joyously thank my soul mate, my husband, and beloved father to all our girls. You listened, helped, and had tremendous patience and understanding. You encouraged me and stood by me every step of the way. Every path and every challenge we endure makes our bond tighter. I am so blessed and thankful for your unconditional love, which we have shared for over thirty-two years.

To Ryan and Corey, your strength, love, and understanding meant everything to us and to Taylor. Without you, Taylor would not have been able to endure her battle in the manner she did. You always had her back, and she knew it. You showered Taylor with the unconditional love that only sisters can share. Thank you for allowing me to share our personal story.

To my dad, my mom, and my twin brother, Paul: love begins at home and never ends. You taught Taylor what love was all about. Andrea, Bill, Samantha, and Sofia, where do I begin? You went to all ends of the earth to help Taylor during her journey. Your love sustained us. You gave Taylor hope, and most important, she knew you were there for her no matter what. Your love and support got me through the unimaginable and helps me live today.

Annie (and yes, I am calling you Annie instead of Andrea), you brought Taylor love and laughs throughout and during her final days. You held us tightly when we lost our daughter. There are no words to ever begin to express our gratitude. Your inspiration, dedication, and passion to tell Taylor's story with me made this book possible. You gave me the strength to persevere and love to support me. You were right by my side, little sis.

To our friends, I am sincerely appreciative for your endless support and the many gifts of love you bestowed on Taylor and our family. You helped Taylor live life on her own terms, always eager to engage with her and share her life-loving energy. Your generosity catapulted our lives. You have become our family.

A round of applause to all of Taylor's friends—thank you for your loving friendships, your laughter, and for playing along with Taylor in her endless adventures. You gave her the normalcy she so deeply craved. You were always there for her no matter what the circumstances, and she counted on it. Taylor and our family are eternally grateful for each of you.

Beata, without the love and tenderness you showed our family every single day, we would not have made it. Thank you for filling my shoes and loving my three daughters, even at your own expense. There are no words of gratitude that would suffice.

I am so grateful to Taylor's medical team for the special bond that each of you had with her. Thank you for collaborating with each other to give Taylor the best treatment options. Taylor trusted you with her life, felt safe in your hands, and knew you were on her team.

Anne, I am beholden to you for your unending encouragement, support, approval, resources, and love for Taylor and me. This memoir would not have been possible without you. The generosity of your heart is astounding.

Thank you to Morgan James Publishing and all the members of their team who made this memoir possible. We greatly appreciate your assistance, guidance, and support and for believing in me. I am forever thankful.

To Amanda, our editor, we thank you for your skill, thorough review of the manuscript, and compassion for my story. Thank you for getting to know Taylor.

Thank you to my fellow "life writers" and my professor, for your guidance and encouragement and for believing in me. I will forever cherish our friendships.

To our superintendent Nancy, I am so grateful for the compassion you gave to both Taylor and our family and for fulfilling Taylor's greatest wishes: to be a normal kid and attend school when possible. You gave her the flexibility she craved and let her live life without academic pressure.

To all of Taylor's teachers, I thank you for giving Taylor the gift of learning much more than a textbook could ever teach her. One of her greatest wishes was to attend school, a tribute to all of you. You made school a stress-free and enriching place for Taylor.

Cheers to our donors. Your continued support, generosity, and personal commitment have made Taylor's wishes, hopes, and dreams eternal. Thank you for helping us save the lives of children with cancer.

About the Authors

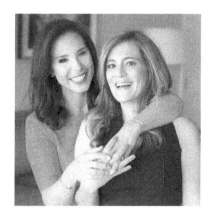

S ue Matthews is the president of the Taylor Matthews Foundation, a nonprofit dedicated to raising awareness and funding pediatric cancer research. She is actively involved in advocating for children with cancer and lobbying Congress for legislation to improve access to cancer treatments for children. Sue navigated hospital systems all across the United States and internationally. She speaks with compassion and detailed knowledge about the options and challenges families face. She holds a BA in accounting from Franklin and Marshall College and is a CPA and former senior manager at Deloitte. Sue lives in New York City with her family.

Andrea Cohane is a board member, advocate, and advisor for her niece Taylor's pediatric cancer foundation. She holds a BS in economics from Cornell University and a Juris Doctorate from Fordham University School of Law. She has practiced business litigation, both in New York City and Charlotte, North Carolina, and is a member of the bar in both states. Andrea resides in Charlotte, with her husband Bill and their children, Samantha and Sofia.

About the Taylor Matthews Foundation

Aportion of the author's proceeds from the sale of this book will be donated to TAY-BANDZ INC., doing business as the Taylor Matthews Foundation.

The Taylor Matthews Foundation, a tay-bandz organization, is a 501(c)(3) nonprofit organization dedicated to raising awareness and funding pediatric cancer research. We fund innovative research and treatments that can reach sick children today, not months or years from now, to improve outcomes and reduce the long-term survivorship side effects associated with pediatric cancer.

For more information, please visit taylormatthewsfoundation.org

If you would like to make a donation of any size, please go to taylormatthewsfoundation.org.

All funds raised go directly to pediatric cancer research.

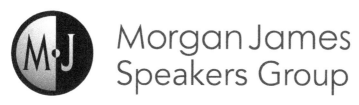

Morgan James
Speakers Group

www.TheMorganJamesSpeakersGroup.com

We connect Morgan James published authors with live and online events and audiences who will benefit from their expertise.

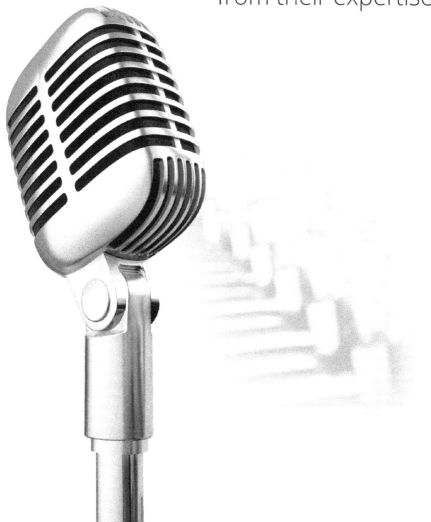

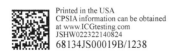

Printed in the USA
CPSIA information can be obtained
at www.ICGtesting.com
JSHW022322140824
68134JS00019B/1238

9 781683 507277